Praise for *Your Everyday Nutrition*

"This book is packed with helpful answers to countless eating questions. Ilyse and Hallie do an exceptional job of providing practical advice with an entertaining dose of humor. You'll laugh, learn, and likely pass on a number of these useful gems to friends and family members!"

—Joy Bauer MS, RDN Founder of Nourish Snacks, #1 *New York Times* bestselling author and NBC's *TODAY Show* nutritionist

"A great read with easy to digest, extremely helpful information on health and nutrition. In a breezy, playful style, Ilyse and Hallie give you useful ideas that you can implement today."

—Joel Harper, NYC Celebrity Fitness Trainer

"I love their approach to health and nutrition. This book gives me the power to make informed decisions in a balanced and achievable way."

—Angie Everhart, model and actress

"The world of nutrition is continually evolving; however, many people are walking around believing information from twenty or thirty years ago. *Your Everyday Nutrition* debunks popular myths and gives you the most up-to-date nutrition and lifestyle information that is relatable and easy-to-understand. It's also a great conversation starter—after reading it, you'll be the one telling family and friends the real deal about many common misconceptions."

—Toby Amidor, MS, RD, national nutrition expert, author of *The Greek Yogurt Kitchen* and columnist for *Today's Dietitian* magazine

Your Everyday Nutrition

100 Answers to the Most Common
Questions about Losing Weight,
Feeling Great, and Getting Healthy

ILYSE SCHAPIRO, MS, RDN
& HALLIE RICH

Foreword by Michelle Beadle

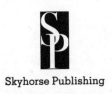

Skyhorse Publishing

Skyhorse Publishing books may be purchased in bulk at special discounts for sales promotion, corporate gifts, fund-raising, or educational purposes. Special editions can also be created to specifications. For details, contact the Special Sales Department, Skyhorse Publishing, 307 West 36th Street, 11th Floor, New York, NY 10018 or info@skyhorsepublishing.com.

Skyhorse® and Skyhorse Publishing® are registered trademarks of Skyhorse Publishing, Inc.®, a Delaware corporation.

Visit our website at www.skyhorsepublishing.com.

10 9 8 7 6 5 4 3 2 1

Library of Congress Cataloging-in-Publication Data is available on file.

Cover design by Kai Texel

Print ISBN: 978-1-5107-7725-5
Ebook ISBN: 978-1-5107-7726-2

Printed in the United States of America

With all our love:
Riley, Perri, Marlene and Bob
Mike, Mason, Mackenzie, Ronni, and Barrie

With loving memory:
Mel Rich, Shelley Schachter, and Shanna Joseph

Disclaimer

The content in this book is designed to provide information and education on the subjects discussed, and it is not a substitute for professional medical advice. Recommendations in this book represent the opinions of Ilyse Schapiro and Hallie Rich and are based upon their knowledge, experience, research, and training. This material has not been reviewed by the US Food and Drug Administration. This book is not meant to be used, nor should it be used, to diagnose or treat any medical condition. Before starting any new program or dietary supplement product, you should consult with your physician or health-care professional, especially if you are taking any medications or have a specific health issue, concern, or problem. The publisher and authors are not responsible for any specific health or allergy needs that may require medical supervision and are not liable for any damages or negative consequences from any treatment, action, application, or preparation to any person reading or following the information in this book. References are provided for informational purposes only and do not constitute endorsement of any products, websites, or other sources.

Please note: The brand names mentioned throughout this book are registered properties of their manufacturers.

Although the authors and publisher have made every effort to ensure that the information in this book was correct at press time, the authors and publisher do not assume and hereby disclaim any liability to any party for any loss, damage, or disruption caused by errors or omissions, whether such errors or omissions result from negligence, accident, or any other cause.

Contents

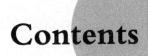

SECTION 2:
THE INSIDE SCOOP ON A HEALTHY LIFESTYLE

SECTION 3:
THE INSIDE SCOOP ON WELLNESS

Foreword
by Michelle Beadle
Former Host of ESPN's *SportsNation*

I don't know about you, but I've reached critical mass in the "miracle cures" department of healthy living. A day doesn't go by that I'm not bombarded with a seemingly endless stream of diets, cleanses, skin care products, and pills that all promise to give me a supermodel body and rock star lifestyle with minimal effort. I've tried it all—every diet, every supplement, and every trick to try to fool the scale. News flash: it ain't happening.

As part of the proverbial rat race, which is hardest on women, there is a constant quest to achieve aesthetic perfection. In my world, I'm judged constantly. Just recently, I gained a few pounds and my "friends" on Twitter let me hear it. You don't think I knew already? I was there when I devoured my guac and chips and the fried chicken and biscuits without hitting the gym.

I may be around celebrities and athletes constantly, but that doesn't mean that I don't stand in front of the mirror and see how I don't always look like them. That's the real world, though. Sometimes we're thinner and other times thicker. Sometimes we're healthier and other times not so much. I know without a trainer, a chef, a makeup artist, and a nutritionist on staff that I'm not always going to look like those I interview. Unless you won the genetic lottery (the actual lottery is more likely), then no amount of carb-cutting or gluten elimination is going to transform me, or you, into Giselle. And that's okay. Even Giselle has issues, right? I mean, there must be something. Watery eyes? Long toes? Anything!

We're all juggling careers, family, and relationships, but tearing ourselves apart in the process has to stop. *Your Everyday Nutrition* has taken every aspect of this circus and broken it down to its core, leaving a succinct and achievable guidebook for overall improvement. What I love about this book is that Ilyse and Hallie know the trends that sucker us in—and they know where these trends may ultimately lead. In a logical, funny, and lighthearted way, they show us how to lead a healthy lifestyle by doing it the right way. Throughout the book, they warmly welcome us in, offer us a nice cup of green tea, and give it to us straight as they explain it all. And *nothing* is off limits.

Without ruining the ending of the book, you know what can work? A realistic approach to what we put in our mouths. It's in the title! How much easier can it be? But it's so much more than that. You already know a pound of bagels a day may lead to a new wardrobe every month (and the not-so-fun kind of shopping with your girlfriends). But who amongst us mere mortals has the willpower to turn down breads? Bread is a beautiful art to be enjoyed. These women allow us the pleasure—hell, they even throw in a schmear—and they do it in a way that doesn't guilt us into shameful closet carb consumption, but rather a way to enjoy yeasty goodness in moderation.

That's the beauty of this book. It's a real way to live a real life. Whether they're discussing sugar, chocolate, sushi, juicing, chia seeds, vitamins, or even sex, there's nothing extreme about their approach. It's amazing how much they can cover while being logical, funny, and lighthearted. You hardly realize you're learning since you feel like you're having a great conversation with friends (who actually know what they're talking about). There are no judgements. They offer friendly advice told through expert eyes and voices. And, they get it.

This book is not like any of the other health, diet, or nutrition books you've read before. Let me clarify that—the books that you've *bought* before. If you're like me, you've purchased more of these books than you know what to do with, but you have either gotten bored midway through the first few sentences, had a hard time finishing it, or felt totally uninspired to do anything it recommends. Even though the subject matter might have been extremely interesting and important, if the delivery isn't there, the book gets slammed shut. Message forever interrupted.

Once you're done "scooping out your bagel," you'll have attainable, realistic, and solid information that will lend itself to all aspects of your life. Hallie and Ilyse break it all down and give us the raw facts, from foods to supplements. Even though I had my nose in this book and read it from cover to cover, I couldn't help but notice the breath of fresh air I experienced each time I turned the page. There are no more reasons to be duped or to feel guilty. They know life is meant to be enjoyed, and they show us the healthy and balanced way to achieve this without sacrificing too much.

Whether you're looking to lose a few pounds or just trying to see if you're on the right path to a healthy lifestyle, these ladies will open your eyes on how to do so. You will never again fall for the smoke and mirrors, as they charmingly bring us behind the curtains and expose a number of secrets. Hallie and Ilyse give it to you straight without leaving you with only (organic) lettuce to munch on. After reading this book, you won't be hungry—or disappointed.

So grab a bagel with schmear, sit back, and get ready to laugh and learn as you get the inside scoop and a brand new outlook.

Introduction

Your *Everyday Nutrition* gives no-holds-barred answers to the questions that keep every modern woman wondering why her weight is high, her libido is low, and her mind is scattered. While many women only feel comfortable asking these types of questions of their best friend, they really desire expert advice. That's where we come in!

As a registered dietitian and a health-industry expert, we are Dear Abby meets *Sex and the City* meets Dr. Oz. Based on our twenty-five years of combined experience in the health field, we are able to cover a multitude of topics constantly at the top of your mind. We cover everything from food and nutrition, to diet and weight loss, as well as healthy habits for the kitchen, bedroom, boardroom, and even the bathroom—nothing is off limits!

Throughout this book, you'll find expert secrets and the tricks of our respective trades. With so much information and so many "rules" out there, we aim to give you the tools to sort through the BS and to know what is truly important and actually relevant to your life. It's normal to feel inundated by all of the information from traditional media, the web, and social media; it's totally understandable to become confused by the information overload and the contradictory messages.

As professionals, we were even more exasperated when we read two recent reports: one by the Institute of Medicine that stated nearly half of all American adults (approximately 90 million people) have difficulty understanding and using health information, and another study that stated 68 percent of Americans agreed with the following statement: "when reporting medical and health news, the media often contradict themselves, so I don't know what to believe" (as cited in Stahl, 2000, p.1298). All of these facts combined were the impetus for us to write this book—it was finally time to set the record straight.

In our consultations, seminars, lectures, and conversations, women constantly come to us to seek clarity over these unending contradictions. In an effort to turn these discussions into a handbook for all matters relating to health, food, and diet, *Your Everyday Nutrition* was born.

Our goal is to answer the questions we get asked repeatedly (whether in professional or personal settings), making sure to keep it light and entertaining. We aim to have you put healthy food in your belly, insightful information in your head, and a smile on your face—all the while making you LOL.

We didn't want to create yet another typical diet or health book. Those books address these topics in an aspirational way and assume people can and will follow all the rules (which they rarely do). Instead, we want to provide you with advice based in reality that can easily be adapted to everyday life. Since you are all extremely busy, we made sure our book is written in a way that is not overwhelming, but rather maximizes your time. Whether you have ample free time on a vacation, only a few minutes while you're waiting in the carpool line or commuting to work, or relishing your precious few private moments alone in the bathroom, *Your Everyday Nutrition* can be read in part or all at once. The book's Q&A format enables you to jump in and out as you please and easily find the subjects you relate to most.

While we take the content seriously, we can't say the same about ourselves. We pride ourselves on being sassy and candid, but we make sure to answer each health question without being patronizing or dictating. We know you will crave dessert, want to dine out, consume alcohol, forget to take your vitamins, and have (with any luck) plenty of sex. We also know you're going to have questions about all of the above. (Who doesn't?!) While there are no "stupid questions," there are plenty of "stupid answers" percolating all around.

We combined our knowledge from the field, with the latest studies and research, to make sure *Your Everyday Nutrition* becomes your trusted health companion. We hope that once you have read this book, not only will you have a better understanding of eating and living well, but that you will also say to yourself, "Who knew scooping out my bagel could be this life changing?"

The Inside Scoop on Nutrition

"Never eat more than you can lift."
—Miss Piggy

1. Should I scoop out my bagel?

Round and thick . . . No, this isn't that kind of book! We're talking about what you'll look like if you eat too many bagels. Scooping a bagel can be extremely helpful if you're trying to eat healthy. By eliminating the dough on the inside and just leaving the shell, you save calories while still getting to enjoy the best part of the bagel. After toasting, it can be even tastier for those of you who like it hard. Wait; it's still not that kind of book!

Bagels tend to be low in fiber and protein and very high in carbs and sodium—not exactly the ingredients for a slim body. So, scooping a bagel won't leave you missing anything important, but it will help you cut excess calories and carbs—but only if you throw out the dough you scooped. Don't nibble on it. Just put it right in the garbage before it tempts you.

Once the bagel is scooped, you have to be careful not to fill the hollowed out bagel with too much "stuff." Pay close attention to the amount you're using and don't bulk up on spreads, salads, or meats. Half of a cup of low-fat tuna, one to two tablespoons of peanut/nut butter, or a couple slices of cheese are appropriate portion sizes and will help fill you up. You can also make a pizza bagel or a sandwich with eggs/egg whites, turkey, or grilled chicken. All of these fillings and options can provide you with nutrients, protein, and/or fiber, which are missing from most bagels. If you can't imagine having a bagel without cream cheese, try to stick to the low-fat or whipped varieties or don't use too much of the full-fat variety at a time. To make it even more exciting, add smoked salmon and lox; they're a great source of omega-3s, vitamin D, and protein. Just beware of their sodium content if salt is a problem for you.

In social or professional situations, if you're too embarrassed to scoop your bagel because you're afraid of how that will look to a date, a boss, or "judgy" friends, try to eat half the bagel and limit the schmear.

If scooping a bagel leaves you feeling empty in the middle, fill the void with mini-bagels, bagel thins, or deli flats. These all have approximately 100 calories as opposed to a "real" bagel which can have at least 300 calories. The packaged bagels in the grocery store can also be an alternative since they usually have half the calories of the freshly baked ones. The taste may not compare, but we love our asses in our favorite jeans more, which sometimes helps when deciding what type of bagel to eat. Be careful, though—read the ingredients and try to avoid those that contain high-fructose corn syrup and lots of preservatives. Also take note of the sodium levels; compare brands and look for ones with the lowest levels (aim for 250 to 375 milligrams per bagel).

Regardless of how you eat your bagel, it's always best to limit the number you eat to one per week since they are dense and have a lot of calories. Try, if possible, to choose 100 percent whole wheat and skip cinnamon raisin and other sweet flavor bagels. Otherwise, the different varieties of bagels are pretty much within range of each other, so pick your favorite kind. As a treat, an entire bagel once in a while won't kill you, but if you indulge more often, it might kill bathing suit season!

2. Why can't I stop eating the bread from the bread basket?

The bread basket is magnetic and turns our nicely manicured hands into monster-like claws. As soon as the waiter or waitress comes by with it, the conversation stops and all eyes are transfixed on the bread. This "carb trap" seems to always hit the table in slow motion, but most people can't get their hands on it fast enough.

This magnetic force isn't really your fault. Since the bread basket at most restaurants tends to be filled with white bread, there's barely any fiber in it. They're basically putting a huge amount of sugar in front of you, which is why it's so addictive. How many of you have said, "I'll just have five jelly beans," which turns into fifty and suddenly you can't stop eating them? It's the same with the evil bread basket. You have a quick fix, your blood sugar spikes, and then when you crash, you crave more.

Here are a few tried-and-true tips that will help stop you from gaining a baker's dozen by the end of the meal!

- Don't eat out of the bread basket. Instead, put a slice of bread on your plate. People tend to eat less when they are more aware of how much they are eating. If you just pick at the rolls in the basket, you're more likely to overindulge and lose count of how much you have eaten. This will make it much harder to know when it's time to stop.
- If you're going to have a slice of bread, use olive oil instead of globbing on butter. It's not only a healthier option, but a little bit goes a long way. Try to put only a small amount of olive oil on your bread plate and don't repour.
- Eat slowly. Take a bite, chew, and take a break. Give your body time to realize it's getting food. Otherwise, you will probably inhale half the basket and get full before you even eat the food you came to the restaurant to try. Rarely, if ever, do you pick a restaurant based on their bread basket. So use caution and save room for the food you came to eat in the first place.
- Don't go into a meal overly hungry. If you do, you will be much more likely to stuff your face with the bread.
- Order an appetizer. If you're hungry and your stomach is growling and you must "get food into your belly," then consider a starter. House salads, vegetable soup, shrimp cocktail, and tuna tartar are great options. You can also start with a

side dish, like sautéed or steamed spinach or another veggie. It is always better to eat nutritiously than to consume empty calories like plain white bread.

- If you simply can't resist, tell them not to put the bread basket down on the table, or just take one piece and have them take the rest away.

3. Should I blot my pizza?

As the pizza cools and you wait to take the first bite without burning the roof of your mouth, the question "to blot or not to blot?" may cross your mind. Do you take the pile of paper napkins and turn them into squares of orange grease, or do you just say "fuggadaboutit" and dig in?

The grease you soak up only adds about 20 to 50 calories per slice. This is pretty negligible if you're just having one slice. You can easily burn off those 20 to 50 calories just by parking a little bit further from the restaurant. Besides, if the pizza has been sitting there for a while, you may not even be soaking up the grease—sometimes what you pick up is just some moisture from the pizza anyway.

Pizza is pizza, and if you can keep it to a slice and you don't have it frequently, there's no reason it can't be enjoyed as-is. If you are looking to keep your weight in check, or if you eat pizza regularly, focus on skipping fatty toppings such as pepperoni, sausage, and extra cheese. Sicilian, white sauce pizza, and specialty slices like breaded chicken and baked ziti should be saved for special occasions. Salad pizza is not necessarily a healthier option either as it is usually drenched in dressing. If you like it, go for it, but don't have it if you're just trying to save calories. The healthiest slices are topped with veggies such as peppers, mushrooms, spinach, or tomatoes. Not only will you be getting some nutrients and saving a ton of fat, but the fiber will help fill you up so you can stick to one slice!

Another way to make your pizza healthier is to order whole wheat. If you want to trick yourself into feeling like you're eating a lot of pizza without actually doing so, cut the slice in half and have two or three small slices. Even better, buy your own whole wheat crust and make a pie of your own at home. This way, you can use healthier tomato sauces, fresh toppings, and limit the oil. Don't be afraid to experiment and try new and exciting recipes for pizza crusts using cauliflower, eggplant, or zucchini. It's okay to make a mistake since, it's been said, pizza is like sex . . . even when it's bad, it's still good!

4. **I'm trying to lose weight. Do I have to give up pasta?**

Mamma Mia! Instead of deciding between popular shapes like penne, ziti, or spaghetti, now it's the *type* of pasta that has us wavering. While regular white pasta is always delicious, it is not the most nutritious, which is why so many people are now looking at alternatives. For traditional pasta, try 100 percent whole wheat pasta. Compared with regular white noodles, it has more fiber, vitamins, and nutrients, plus you will get all the benefits of eating whole grains. Pair it with a veggie and add some protein to help you limit the quantity (stick to one serving) and also to help to keep you more satisfied. Other healthy substitutions to try are spaghetti squash, brown rice pasta, noodles made from soba or shirataki, or pasta made from zucchini or hearts of palm. Don't be fooled by boxed pasta enriched with vegetables, as it is usually deceiving. These generally add color to your bowl of pasta, but not nutrients. As for chickpea pasta, while it may be higher in protein, it still has a substantial amount of carbs, meaning you still need to be mindful and watch the portion size. The same thing goes for gluten-free pasta. These products are not necessarily healthier either; they can still be high in carbs and fat. Make sure to not fall for marketing terms—turn over the box and read all labels.

Quinoa and kaniwa are also great and healthy options. Although technically seeds, they are treated more like a grain. While kaniwa is crunchier and less bitter, in many ways they are very similar to each other: they are both high in protein, fiber, iron, and are gluten free. They both cook quickly, which is a great thing for anyone preparing a meal in a hurry (I think that includes most of us!). You can also use the leftovers for salads and soups, or as a substitute for oatmeal, rice, risotto, or potatoes.

Farro, on the other hand, is a grain. It is high in protein, fiber, and iron, while also containing zinc. It can be higher in fat and calories, but you're also getting more nutrients, so it's still considered a healthier alternative than traditional white pasta. Farro can be very filling, which means it automatically helps with portion control. While a bit less nutritious, bulgur contains many of the same beneficial properties as farro. It also contains fewer calories and grams of fat.

5. **Whole wheat, seven grain, rye, oh my! What is the healthiest bread to eat?**

It's no wonder many of us have moved away from plain white bread since it really has no nutritional value. The question then becomes, which bread does? Any way you slice it, there are lots of traps, so before you spend your dough, be sure to take these things into consideration:

Multigrain breads contain multiple types of grains (obviously!) and they're meant to sound healthier than white bread. However, that's not necessarily true. It's not the number of grains that matter, but the type. If the first ingredient in your loaf of bread is enriched bleached flour, enriched wheat flour, or wheat flour, you're mostly eating white flour—regardless of whether it's seven grain or twelve grain.

Instead of buying bread based on how many grains it has, look at the label and find one whose first ingredient is 100 percent whole wheat, 100 percent whole grain, whole wheat, or whole wheat flour. This ensures you're getting the benefits, including more fiber and nutrients and less refined flour. Otherwise, there's only a grain of truth to your bread being a lot healthier than white bread.

Be careful of the terms *wheat bread*, *100% wheat*, or *enriched wheat*. These terms only mean they originated from wheat flour, but they don't tell you how the bread was manufactured. If the grains are processed, it may destroy the nutrients and any advantages you thought it had over white flour.

Rye bread can be a good choice, as it is high in fiber and doesn't normally result in a spike of your blood sugar. This can help you stay fuller for longer and you will be less likely to find yourself in a bread coma.

No matter the type of bread you choose, be mindful that most contain a ton of sodium. For example, even a slice of 100 percent whole wheat bread can have 150 milligrams of sodium. That's more than an order of small fries from McDonald's. This doesn't mean you should be rushing out to get fast food instead of having a sandwich; it just means you should be aware of other sources of sodium in your diet and choose your bread wisely.

When selecting a loaf, try to avoid those with high-fructose corn syrup, caramel, molasses, and other sweeteners or colors that are usually added to disguise the look and taste of bread.

6. Are wraps the sandwich solution?

When wraps first came out, everyone thought they were the answer to their diet needs. They were thinner, flatter, and some were even made with vegetables, so it was easy to believe they were healthier. However, just like the guy who was hot in his profile picture but looked much different in person, everything isn't always as it seems.

Wraps can actually be higher in calories than regular sliced bread. They can also have twice as many carbs and higher levels of sodium. Wraps usually contain a type of trans fat called partially hydrogenated oils. Even the ones supposedly made of spinach and tomato are often misleading, as these vegetables are added primarily for color and seasoning instead of for their nutritional value. If you're really looking to get spinach and tomato into your diet, your best bet is to put them in the wrap as part of your sandwich. That's the only way to guarantee you're getting their essential nutrients.

The unhealthiest part of the wrap is usually the abundance of stuff in the middle. Wraps tend to be very bulky and overflowing, and there is no need for that much turkey, tuna, roast beef, breaded chicken, or egg salad. They also usually have lots of toppings and fillings, like creamy dressings, mayo, cheese, and bacon.

These mouth-watering wraps don't always need to be gut-busting disasters if you stick to lean meats with veggies. If it's a pre-made wrap, and it's overly full, try to only eat half—it should be more than enough to fill you up. You can also save calories by avoiding the foldings at each end of the wrap. This is just extra bread, empty calories, and unnecessary additional carbs.

To make wraps as healthy as possible, pick 100 percent whole wheat if it's available; they are higher in fiber and more nutritious. Additionally, try to prepare these sandwiches at home so you can be in control of what's in them. Pick wraps that are 100 calories or fewer. Or, you can get creative with sandwiches and use lettuce leaves, portabella mushrooms, or even eggplant to hold it together instead of bread. And that's a wrap on wraps!

7. What's the healthiest breakfast cereal?

Ever look disapprovingly at someone in the grocery store as they put Fruit Loops in their shopping cart while you put Smart Start in yours? Especially with a name like Smart Start, you think it's so much healthier, right? Wrong! Fruit Loops has 12 grams of sugar, while Smart Start actually has 14 grams of sugar for the same serving size (1 cup). While they both have the same amount of fiber (3 grams), Smart Start has half the fat (0.5 grams to 1 gram) but 80 more calories per serving (190 calories to 110 calories). Your choice isn't better after all.

While we tend to think most sugary and unhealthy cereals come in crazy colors and are marketed toward kids, that's just not the case anymore. Even though many brands might imply they're good for you, it's important to turn the boxes over and look at the ingredients to see what they're really made of and from. You'd be shocked! Nutrition facts don't lie. Start with grams of sugar. To think that Raisin Bran and Kashi Go Lean Crunch have more sugar than Cinnamon Toast Crunch and Frosted Mini Wheats might seem crazy—but it's true!

If you really want to make your head spin, take a look at the serving size. Bear Naked Fruit & Nutty Granola, for example, only has 7 grams of sugar, but the serving size is ¼ cup. If you had a full cup of this, which is a pretty normal portion, you would be consuming 28 grams of sugar! Get ready for a sugar high. More to the point, don't assume that all brands have the same serving size. Regular Cheerios has a serving size of 1 cup, but Honey Nut Cheerios has a serving size of ¾ cup. Additionally, while both are marketed as high protein, keto-friendly, and "healthier" alternatives, Cocoa Magic Spoon's serving size is 1 cup while Catalina Crunch Dark Chocolate Cereal is ½ cup. They're all probably counting on the fact that you don't want to do math with fractions to compare and contrast like you had to do in school!

After you've seen the serving size, check out the ingredients. Even if your favorite box of cereal is splashed with MADE WITH WHOLE GRAIN on the front of the box, if it doesn't say 100 percent whole grain in the ingredient section, then it's probably not made with that much. Don't stop there, though. Look for artificial sweeteners, flavors, and food dyes. Even those cereals that you wouldn't see advertised on Saturday morning cartoons may contain them. Fiber 1 has aspartame, Quaker Oatmeal Squares uses yellow #5, and Special K Vanilla Almond contains artificial flavors.

Lastly, don't get stuck on fiber. While it would be ideal to get 3 or more grams of fiber per 1-cup serving, it's not the only factor when buying cereal. You can always add fruit to your cereal or on the side and get natural fiber that way. The same is true with protein. Incorporate nuts, flaxseeds, or hard-boiled eggs into your breakfast.

However, cereal isn't a total lost cause. There are some good options out there, including Cheerios, Barbara's Puffins, Kashi Heart to Heart, and All Bran Complete Wheat Flakes. When you're shopping, you have to be educated. Don't only look at calories and fat, look at the big picture. All of the information on a cereal box is important, don't just judge it by the cover.

8. Lately, it seems there are so many types of milk. What's the difference?

Holy cow! It's easy to get overwhelmed by the sheer number of cartons to choose from in the dairy section. Between cows' milk and plant-based milks (like almond, rice, soy, and flax), it's udder chaos. (We know, we know.)

Which one is best? It's really up to you! Cows' milk has more protein than any of the plant-based milks and contains more vitamins and minerals. It's a natural source of complete protein, meaning it contains all nine essential amino acids and is also high in calcium, vitamin D, and vitamin A. Goats' milk is also a great source of these nutrients, and has the added benefits of being easy to digest and containing less lactose. Whichever you prefer, you have to pay special attention to the fat and calorie contents. Whole milk has the most fat and calories, reduced-fat (2%) and low-fat milk (1%) obviously fall in the middle, and skim/nonfat milk has the least.

Plant-based milks also contain many vitamins and minerals (like A, B2, B12, and D), but their nutritional benefits depend on their source. Soy milk is a good source of protein and has the highest amount compared to other plant-based milks. Almond milk, rice milk, and flax milk tend to be lower in protein but have other benefits; they can be fortified with calcium and vitamin D and low in saturated fats and cholesterol. Flax milk has the added benefit of containing omega-3s. Hemp milk is also a great alternative to cows' milk. It's rich in many vitamins and minerals and also in omega-3s. Sorry to disappoint, though—it won't give you a high. Oat milk, while a popular non-dairy milk, may be a good alternative for those who have dairy and nut allergies or sensitivities. However, it is higher in carbohydrates and calories than other plant-based milks and can have added oils to thicken it, so be mindful to check ingredients if you're watching your weight.

Many of these plant-based milks come in flavored forms that have loads of sugar and artificial additives. Even the deceptively innocent "original" or "plain" versions can contain added sugars. Make sure to look at the ingredients and the nutrition panel. A glass of chocolate plant-based milk can have the same amount of sugar as a handful of cookies or a chocolate bar.

No matter the source, as long as you're mindful of calories, fat, and added sugar, there's no point crying over spilled milk as long as you're a smart cookie.

9. **How can I get my cheese fix in a healthy way?**

Cheese is one of those things that you can like whether it's soft or hard. From melted mozzarella to blocks of cheddar, cheese can be so delicious that Wisconsin isn't the only home to cheeseheads.

Cheese can be a great snack or addition to a meal, as it is normally high in calcium and protein. It can also contain other nutrients including vitamins A and B12, phosphorous, and zinc. The National Dairy Council recommends Swiss, cheddar, ricotta, mozzarella, Monterey Jack, and Gouda as the most nutritious cheeses.

Even though some cheeses tend to be high in fat and sodium, the yummiest cheeses need not be avoided. Since their flavors are very powerful, a few bites will leave you happy and satisfied. A little bit of good cheese can go a long way. Alternatively, if you go for the less-flavorful varieties, you may not get the fix you wanted and end up nibbling on way more cheese than you intended.

Beware of alternatives in the dairy aisle, especially if you're not a cheese connoisseur. Avoid the no-fat options; many contain fillers and preservatives, and the taste can be worse than any cheesy joke. They also are not ideal for cooking. Instead, look for those products that use low-fat milk or are part skim and are lower in sodium.

While cheese seems pretty easy to identify, there are those that should not even qualify as part of the category. Some of the

An Extra Scoop!

If you've stayed away from cheese because of a lactose intolerance or sensitivity, you may not have to stay away from cheese completely. Try hard cheeses like cheddar and Parmesan. During their processing, most of the lactose is removed so only low levels are left.

most popular cheeses aren't even cheese at all. Many American single-sliced cheese products are listed as "pasteurized prepared cheese product," i.e., not really cheese. This can be due to the process it undergoes and the number of fillers and other preservatives and additives it uses. While this isn't necessarily reason enough to avoid them, just bear in mind that a good chunk of the product is not cheese.

Try to stay away from those products that don't resemble cheese. For example, those that come in squeezy tubes, cans, or powders. If you wouldn't use it to trap a mouse, chances are it's not something you really want to be eating a lot of.

10. **What's all the hype with yogurt? It seems all Greek to me!**

Olive oil, feta cheese, and fish aren't the only great foods to come from the Mediterranean region. The Greek gods have continued to bless us with Greek yogurt.

Greek yogurt can be an excellent source of nutrients. Not only does it contain B vitamins, calcium, magnesium, potassium, and phosphorous, but it also has plenty of probiotics.

These nutrients can help with your skin, digestion, stomach, immunity, and even your metabolism (for more information on probiotics, see page 179). Greek yogurt also tends to be high in protein, which can help you feel full and therefore prevent unnecessary snacking or munching.

In terms of flavor, Greek yogurt tends to be a bit more tart than most other yogurts. However, what it may lack in taste, it makes up for in texture, as Greek yogurt has a very smooth and creamy consistency. This can make it great for dips, dressings, as a topping, or even an additional ingredient when cooking. It is also wonderful because it can be used as a substitute in baking for higher fat ingredients like cream cheese, mayo, butter, oil, and even sour cream. By using Greek yogurt, you can cut calories and fat and even boost the protein in some of your favorite dishes or treats.

As with any kind of yogurt, if you buy different flavors, be careful of added sugars. The "fruit on the bottom" variety or the fruit flavors can have more than double the sugar of the plain kind. The best option is always to add your own goodies to plain yogurt, including flaxseeds, walnuts, a teaspoon of jam or honey, or even your favorite fruit. These can help make the taste more desirable and as decadent as you'd like. Also, be careful of those that contain whey protein concentrates, cornstarch, milk protein concentrates, and other thickeners, as these ingredients are common in Greek-style yogurts. True Greek yogurt is mostly milk and live cultures and it doesn't use (or need) these additives because it goes through a stringent straining process.

Greek yogurt can be a godsend if you are sensitive to dairy because it tends to be lower in lactose and easier to digest. It also can be a good source of protein and nutrients if you follow a vegetarian diet. Just don't assume that they are all free of animal products, as some brands add gelatin and other non-vegetarian ingredients.

Greek yogurt helps prove that marathons and the Olympics aren't the only great things we got from the Greeks!

11. Where should I be spreading the love . . . butter or margarine?

Butter may not be as bad as has been widely reported over the past few decades, so there's no reason to feel like a lard if you like it.

Butter is made solely from either cows' milk or cream. It contains vitamins A, D, E, and K, which are good antioxidants and have many of their own benefits. While butter is high in saturated fat, recent studies report that it alone won't necessarily lead to heart disease. If you use butter sparingly and in moderation (on a potato, to cook with, or while baking) and have no major overriding health concerns, you don't need to worry about it. However, if you are the type of person who has a side of bread with their butter, it might be time to think again!

Lean toward whipped butter which, due to the air, is lighter and leaner. This will help you save about half the calories, fat, and cholesterol. Light, low-fat butter, or those combined with oils can be comparable to whipped butter in terms of their nutritional profile. However, they may contain fillers, binders, and other additives to help reduce the fat and calorie counts.

Due to this, some varieties may have a waxier consistency and less of a taste. The lower impact of flavor may cause you to use more, which means you might as well have used the full-fat variety to begin with. You can also look at grass-fed butter as a healthier option as these tend to contain more unsaturated fats and omega-3 fatty acids. If you're choosing vegan butter, be aware of the types of oils used as some may contain high amounts of saturated fats. Vegan butter can also contain lots of "extra" ingredients. If either of these are a concern for you, try olive oil or avocado oil as possible substitutes.

Margarine differs from butter because it is normally plant based and made of vegetable oils. Margarine can be very high in trans fats, which can lead to high levels of bad cholesterol (LDL) and low levels of good cholesterol (HDL). Sticks of margarine are the worst offenders. As margarine isn't naturally solid, it must go through a process of hydrogenation, which creates more trans fats. While the tubs tend to have fewer trans fats, their benefits are still spread thin.

Be wary of sprays, too. While they may seem low in calories, if you use a lot, they won't stay that way for long. Sprays also tend to have a lot of artificial ingredients and flavors to get them to replicate the taste of butter, but they often don't come close to duplicating it.

12. Are egg whites all they're cracked up to be?

The decision to eat egg whites or the whole egg has always been tough to crack. Conventional thinking suggested that egg whites were healthier since this is the part of the egg where the protein is, while the yolk of the egg is loaded with dietary cholesterol that supposedly clogged arteries. However, new research states that the egg yolk may not be as bad for us as initially reported. While the egg yolk can affect your cholesterol level and does have more calories, studies have reported it may not directly affect heart disease. Furthermore, most of the nutrients in the egg are found in the yolk, including vitamins A, E, and K as well as B12, folate, calcium, carotenoids, essential fatty acids, DHA, and amino acids. It is also one of the few foods that naturally contain vitamin D. All these nutrients are very important and are discarded if you only eat the egg whites! In contrast, the benefits of the white are limited to just protein and magnesium. While these are important, they will leave you scrambling for other ways to get all of the goodies you would get from eating the entire egg.

If cholesterol or heart disease isn't an issue for you, you may want to go with the whole egg. You can also always eat a half egg-white omelet and half regular (yellow) egg omelet just to switch things up or cut calories. No matter what type of eggs you prefer, make sure not to be rotten with what else you put on your plate. Try to skip the bacon and home fries and go with fruit or a side salad instead.

Whether you prefer omelets, scrambled, over easy, or poached eggs, you now have free range to do what you think is right for your body.

An Extra Scoop!

Eggs fortified with omega-3s are quickly growing in popularity, but if you still prefer only eating the whites, don't waste your money. To obtain these nutrients, you must eat the entire egg, not just the yolk.

13. **I'd rather spend time in the morning getting ready. What are some quick but healthy breakfast options?**

Mornings are super stressful and busy, as there is only a limited amount of time to get everything done between the time the alarm goes off and the time you have to walk out the door. Whether you're just responsible for getting yourself ready, or if your family depends on you, breakfast sometimes gets missed or overlooked. Here are some easy, nutritious, and quick choices that can help you avoid scrambling for ideas in the morning.

- *Avocado Toast*—A favorite for many because it's so tasty, avocado toast should be made with two slices of whole grain toast with ¼ to ½ of an avocado. This provides a great mix of whole grains, fiber and healthy fats to start the day off right. To jazz it up but still keep it healthy, you can add eggs (like sunny side up or hard boiled), seasonings (like everything but the bagel, pepper flakes, or sea salt), smoked salmon, cucumbers and dill, pumpkin seeds or chia seeds.

- *Bowl of oatmeal*—While old-fashioned, slow-cooked, or steel-cut oats are better for you than a packet of instant oatmeal, all of them can be part of a quick, healthy breakfast. If you prefer the old-fashioned kind that takes more time, you can easily make it the night before, store it in the fridge, and heat it up in the morning. Plain instant oats in a packet are a great runner-up, but be wary of the flavored kind where the sugar can add up. You can always add your own fruit, nuts, or cinnamon for taste too.

- *Yogurt with cereal or fruit*—Yogurt, especially the Greek kind, is packed with protein. Pair it with half a cup of cereal, some berries, or 1 to 2 tablespoons of nuts or chia seeds and you have a quick, easy, no mess, and satisfying breakfast.

- *Toast or whole grain waffle with nut butter*—What better way to start off the morning than with something that makes you feel like a kid! With whole grains from the toast or waffle and protein and healthy fat from the nut butter, you will be happy and full for hours! As an alternative, you can also put your nut butter on an apple or banana.

- *Eggs and toast*—Scrambling eggs only takes a couple of minutes and little oversight. You can have one to two whole eggs, or one egg with two to three whites. Pair that with a piece of whole wheat toast or two whole wheat crisp bread crackers. The combo of protein and good carbs will pack the perfect punch. If you tend to oversleep or can't stand leaving a dirty kitchen, make hard-boiled eggs the night before. Then, in the morning, grab them and go! Try taking out the yolks and filling them with some hummus as a fun alternative.

- **Bowl of cereal with milk**—How easy is this? Pour yourself about 1 cup of cereal. As healthy as some of the non-sugar cereal can be, it gets tricky when you eat too much. Look at the label and aim for those that have about 120 calories per ¾ to 1 cup serving, 3 or more grams of fiber and 8 or less grams of sugar per serving. Use some low-fat milk and pair with some berries or even 1 to 2 tablespoons chopped nuts. Need this on the go? Pour it into a plastic cup and have it with a plastic spoon, or use Tupperware for portability.

14. Don't sugarcoat it. Do I really have to give up sweets?

If you tend to consume a lot of refined sugar, then it's a good idea to cut back. It has been well reported that having a major sweet tooth can lead to weight gain. Whether in ways you can see (like on your waist) or in ways that you can't (like in your liver), this extra bulge can lead to short- and long-term health problems. Too much refined sugar can also lead to aging faster and can get in the way of your body's ability to fight bacteria and viruses.

On labels, look at the sugar content and watch out for "added sugars." If you don't see sugar listed as an ingredient, it doesn't mean it's not there. Words that are used to disguise sugar tend to end in *–ose* like dextrose, fructose, lactose, galactose, glucose, sucrose, and maltose. They also often have the word *syrup* or *juice* in them. Examples include corn syrup, fruit juice concentrate, maple syrup, malt syrup, and cane juice. Other less obvious names for sugar include dextrin, honey, hydrogenated starch, invert sugar, rice malt, nectars, molasses, polyols, and sorghum. With all this new lingo, it's incredibly important to read labels carefully and remember that knowing synonyms isn't just something you had to be mindful of for your SATs. Look at what you buy with a discerning eye and take note of the sugar sources. It's not always obvious that something may be high in sugar. For example, did you know a serving of tomato sauce, granola, dried fruit, or a frozen dinner meal can have the same amount of sugar (or even more) than a serving of sugary morning cereal?

Giving up refined sugar completely can be very difficult since it's extremely addictive. It's hard to quit cold turkey. It can take anywhere from a few weeks to several months to break any bad habit, including eating too many sweets, so start slowly and stay committed. At the same time, be careful not to immediately restrict yourself so much that all you do is think about that candy calling your name. Over time, you have probably rewarded yourself with sweets, so you have to reprogram your thought process. It will take a bit of hard mental work to disassociate the emotional relationship you have had with food. When you get the craving for something sweet, work on changing your routine. Instead of reaching for licorice, go for a piece of fruit that has complex carbs instead. If that won't cut it, stick with a small treat that has fewer than 150 calories.

Sugar doesn't need to be your enemy, as it's pretty unrealistic to expect that you're going to eliminate it all from your diet. There is no reason to set yourself up for disappointment. Just be aware of how much refined sugar you're having since you don't need spoonfuls of sugar to make food go down.

5. **Having ice cream can feel sinful. Should I have frozen yogurt instead, or just stick with the real thing?**

Scoop for scoop, ice cream is usually better. Think of frozen yogurt like a fake designer bag you would buy on a street corner. At first you love it. Then you can't stop staring at its imperfections. Finally, you're mad at yourself for buying it and swear off fake bags forever! Frozen yogurt usually affects you the same way. First you have the craving because it sounds delicious and healthy in your head. Then it hits your mouth and you're not always satisfied. By the time you get home, you're gassy, still hungry, and vow next time you're just going for the real stuff.

There's no reason to have a meltdown, because ice cream isn't a bad choice if you can be happy eating a few spoonfuls without packing on the toppings. Half a cup of regular ice cream is comparable to half a cup of frozen yogurt. Both can be as low as 150 calories—a perfect calorie amount for a treat. Regular vanilla or chocolate ice cream, though, will keep you more satisfied, and you usually don't need all the toppings to enhance the flavor. On the other hand, since frozen yogurt can be full of chemicals and other additives, it can taste artificial.

In these cases, it usually takes chocolate chips, sprinkles, syrups, hot fudge, cookies, nuts, or candy to make it taste the way you want it to. This is especially bad at self-serve shops where you have access to huge cups to fill and all of the yogurt and toppings you want. By the time you get to the register, it's hard to see the yogurt underneath all the stuff you've put on top. This can, at the very least, double the amount of calories and eliminate any hope of it being a low-cal treat.

If you can't resist frozen yogurt, try the new bars made with Greek yogurt (like Yasso bars). These are made with non-fat Greek yogurt so they are higher in protein, which can help you feel more satisfied.

16. Does being a chocoholic have any benefits, or will it just leave me fat and broken out?

Our friends know better than to get between us and chocolate. However, we both know that we have to eat it in moderation, and that when it comes to health benefits, dark chocolate is definitely the way to go. The darker the better, especially if it has 70 percent cocoa content or higher.

Research has shown moderate intake of dark chocolate can help support heart health, blood pressure, LDL cholesterol, and blood sugar. It also contains antioxidants, vitamins, and minerals, which have great benefits for the body. What's more? Some studies have even reported that dark chocolate contains the same chemical your brain creates when you're falling in love—so there's actually a reason chocolate has become a "go-to" gift from your significant other or an even better gift to yourself when you need a pick-me-up. Being in love with chocolate actually makes scientific sense.

If dark chocolate isn't your thing, don't fret. White and milk chocolate may not give you some of the advantages associated with dark chocolate, but let's be honest—you're not going for the chocolate bar because of its potential health benefits. The fact that they may have little to no nutritional value (white chocolate is actually made from cocoa butter, milk, and sugar) means that as long as you are just having a little bit, infrequently and as a treat, there's no reason to freak out.

While too much of any kind of chocolate can be fattening, by itself it does not cause acne. If it is part of an unhealthy and unbalanced diet full of fats and sugars, the chocolate won't help matters and your skin may suffer. Chocolate also isn't the root cause of breakouts during your period. We just tend to crave chocolate around this time so it's usually a coincidence. Your hormones are what's to blame, so if chocolate helps with your PMS, have a bite (not a bar), as a little bit can go a long way.

Even though some may wish chocolate was a food group (including us), chocolate can be guilt free! Just remember that less is more, the darker the better, and enjoy it while it lasts.

7. **What should I do when I'm still hungry after dinner and all I want to do is raid the fridge?**

This is one of those times that you need to have a serious talk with yourself. Say to yourself: "Am I really hungry or am I just bored? Am I just thinking of food because it's a bad habit I've gotten myself into over the years?" Chances are, after a big meal, you're actually not hungry and probably will answer yes to one of the above questions.

If you end up evading your own questions, try drinking a glass of water. Many times, dehydration mimics hunger, so you may actually be mistaking your want for food with your need for liquids. After you have a drink, try waiting a few minutes and distract yourself, then see if you're still hungry. If the urge passes, then you've just saved yourself calories and probably were not hungry to begin with. This may especially be true if you've been out boozing and your body is dehydrated. Too many times on the way home from a long night out, our bodies may think they need a grilled cheese sandwich, a slice of pizza, or a side of fries, but they really just need a glass of water.

If you're still famished, try to figure out why. Before the meal, did you drink too much (juice, alcohol, or soda) or did you fill up on bread? If so, that may have caused you to get stuffed before dinner. This will leave you with loads of empty calories but no real food or nutrients to keep you satisfied, and you will indeed get hunger pains by the time you get home. Next time, try to drink water with your meal and go for a healthier appetizer to avoid this happening again.

In the meantime, you're going to need to eat something because right now you're hungry. If a snack will do and you're only mildly hungry, keep it to a few bites and try to limit the calories to 200 or fewer. If you really are starving because dinner didn't satisfy you, try to eat something light (low-fat yogurt, scrambled eggs, pbj/nut butter sandwich). Try not to resort to fried, greasy, or fast foods and keep the portions in check. You did, in fact, already eat some food, so you shouldn't need a full and caloric second dinner. Regularly eating two dinners is only good for producing two chins!

18. What's the deal with breakfast for dinner?

Once you get out of your day clothes, change into your comfy sweats or PJs, and throw your hair up in a messy bun, breakfast foods can be very tempting. After a long day, it's sometimes hard to get motivated to cook a full dinner. Picking up the phone to order take-out or delivery can also seem like too much work and a waste of money. That's when breakfast can make a great dinner. You just have to make sure it doesn't become an all-you-can-eat breakfast buffet.

Eggs, fruit with cottage cheese, one bowl of cereal with low-fat milk, or toast with peanut butter are all well-balanced options to have at night. Stay away from the sugary cereals, as they can have excess calories and all the sugar can make you crave multiple portions. Frozen whole wheat waffles or pancakes can be fun and delicious and can feel a lot more indulgent than they actually are. Not only can they be low in calories, but they can also be quick and easy to prepare in the toaster. If you like them with syrup, just use a little bit and don't drown them. You can even put the syrup on a separate small plate or bowl, which may help you control the amount you use. Try to pair these waffles or pancakes with some slivered almonds, hard-boiled egg, or fresh fruit to also add some protein, fiber, and nutrients.

The major difference between eating breakfast at night as opposed to in the morning is that you're usually not in a rush to get anywhere. You might be eating dinner while on the phone, watching TV, or just decompressing from a long day. This can sometimes lead to grazing and eating more than you usually would. So be careful of portion sizes and going back for seconds, as breakfast foods tend to be less filling than normal dinner meals.

It's fine to switch up any meal of the day—it's not when you eat what, but what you eat when. You can even have dinner for breakfast. Healthy options in the morning can include salads, soups, chicken, whole wheat pasta, beans, fish, and even a leftover slice of whole wheat pizza. Foods rich in protein, nutrients, healthy fats, and/or fiber will give you the fuel you need to power through your day. Eating breakfast like a king may not be as common in the United States, but it's something worth importing.

19. Can I really eat an endless amount of fruits?

How many people do you know who will tell you they let themselves go because they ate too much fruit? Probably zero. Nobody got fat from having too many fruit salads.

Fruits should be a very important part of your daily diet. Not only are they delicious and refreshing, but they are very nourishing as well. Fruits are high in vitamins, antioxidants, fiber, and water. They have been shown to help with immunity, beauty, and energy and can help lower the risk of cardiovascular disease, blood pressure, and cholesterol. Due to the natural fiber, fruit has also been shown to help maintain a healthy GI tract.

Fruit has sugar, which can add up by the end of each day, so don't go bananas! Unlimited amounts of most things, including fruit, won't necessarily help keep you skinny, as it's not calorie free. However, alone it won't leave you with a pear shape. The fiber should help fill you up, so you really shouldn't be in a position where you're eating too much of it. Just make sure to vary what you eat and, like anything, keep it in check. Have a cup of berries, an apple, some slices of melon, or a handful of grapes as opposed to eating an entire cantaloupe. However, if you're hungry, fruits are a low-calorie, filling, and nutritious option—especially opposed to almost anything else you might grab.

Just because something has the word *fruit* in it doesn't mean it's healthy. A fruit smoothie can have 400 calories, and that's before you factor in other ingredients like yogurt or milk. Dried fruits are usually filled with added sugar and have lots of calories despite their small serving size. Fruit juice may be the worst culprit. Unless it's 100 percent juice, you're most likely getting a glass of sugar and calories. While fruit is part of the cocktail, so are artificial additives, sweeteners, and preservatives. Most fruit juice concentrates are just as unhealthy as soda. Ocean Spray Cran Apple Juice Drink has 31 grams of sugar and Welch's 100% Grape Juice has 36 grams of sugar. We're guessing that's way more sugar than you would have thought!

Stick with what Mother Nature has to offer and aim to eat two to four servings of fruit per day. An apple a day really will help keep the doctor away and your weight at bay.

20. **Since peanut butter has been outlawed in so many places, what's a good and healthy alternative?**

Food allergies can be very serious, and it's not nuts for certain households, schools, and organizations to ban them. As nut allergies continue to become more prevalent, so do nut-free options.

If you are allergic to only peanuts, but all other nuts are okay, there are plenty of choices. Think of your favorite nut, and there is probably a spread made from it. There's almond butter, cashew butter, macadamia nut butter, and walnut butter. Nutritionally, these all have relatively the same amount of calories and fat as peanut butter, and they also contain vitamins, minerals, antioxidants, and omega-3 fatty acids. While the tastes may be a little different, some people actually prefer them. For others, once they've gotten used to it, they learn to love them too.

You can also try those that combine fruit and nuts. These can make any lunch or snack even more exciting and may give you the rich flavor you were looking for. Make sure to read labels, as many brands can be high in sugar and carbs and are better suited as a treat instead of as part of a meal.

If you have to avoid all nuts, then you might want to try sunflower butter, pumpkin butter, or pea butter. Soy butter and tahini are great choices as well, but since they are made from soy and sesame seeds respectively, they may be problematic, as these are also top allergens.

Here are some tips when trying out a new spread:

- Don't assume they are all pure blends. Some almond butters, for example, also contain cashews, pine nuts, brazil nuts, and macadamia nuts. Watch the ingredients and check the label.
- Be careful of added sugars, oils, and salt, which can make them unhealthier than the natural versions. Look for no-salt or no-sugar-added varieties wherever possible.
- Watch the serving sizes, as the calories can add up quickly. Be sure not to use too much. The standard serving size is just 2 tablespoons, which can be met and surpassed pretty quickly.
- Get creative in the kitchen and make spreads at home. To limit the preservatives and sugars and other ingredients you may not want, look at recipes online and have fun doing it yourself. It may be a little messy, but with a food processor or blender, it's not that difficult. You can also flavor them to your choosing, which is always nice, especially for picky eaters.

Once you find one(s) that you like, go ahead and use them on sandwiches, apples, and crackers, while you're baking, or even while making a smoothie. Don't be afraid to go nuts(less)!

21. Is Nutella really that bad for me?

Nutella is so attractive to so many of us because it looks like chocolate but feels like something healthy. It's neither. It's actually a hazelnut spread with added cocoa powder. The list of ingredients is fairly short: sugar, palm oil, hazelnuts, cocoa, skim milk, whey, lecithin, and vanillin (an artificial flavor). On the plus side, there are no artificial colors or preservatives, which is great. Nutella is also peanut free, gluten free, kosher, and the palm oil is not hydrogenated, which gives it some more points.

On the other hand, the main ingredients are sugar and oil, which are not great. In fact, one serving is two tablespoons, and this amounts to 200 calories, 21 grams of sugar, and 21 grams of carbs! That's about double the sugar and calories in a serving of Trix Cereal! Mind. Blown.

With Nutella, you're also not getting much protein, so don't kid yourself—having a tablespoon of it is *not* the nutritional equivalent to a handful of hazelnuts. Nutella only has 2 grams of protein per serving. Comparatively, peanut butter has approximately 8 grams of protein (while also having the added benefits of only 2 to 3 grams of sugar and double the fiber). It's not like you're getting any benefits from the cocoa powder since the amount you'd be getting from Nutella is negligible. It's sad to say, but you'd get double the protein with peanut butter M&Ms than you do with Nutella.

If you're looking for a special treat on a Sunday morning, enjoy a serving of Nutella on whole wheat bread or pancakes or spread it on an apple or banana. Keep in mind that there are other options that can provide more health benefits than this faux-chocolate spread. Products like Justin's Chocolate Hazelnut Butter Blend only have 8 grams of sugar per serving and 12 grams of carbs and would make a better choice when you're looking to curb the same type of craving. You could also combine a healthy nut butter with some melted dark chocolate and make your own blend.

With Nutella, since you're not really getting the health benefits of the nuts or the chocolate, you certainly have to "spread the happy" because you're not spreading much else.

22. I'm so confused. Should I be eating sugar-free or fat-free foods?

There is no need to be confused or overwhelmed about this decision. The only thing you should be doing is keeping it real.

The fat-free craze is over. Just like the floppy disc, the DVD player, and mom jeans, eating "fat-less" is a thing of the past. People thought a fat-free diet would be the answer to their prayers. Without fat, how could you not lose weight? It's simple. When fats are removed from food, they usually have to be replaced by something else to ensure that the taste and texture stay the same. That is why fat-free foods usually have added sugar, salt, additives, artificial flavors, sweeteners, and/or preservatives. You end up replacing a known entity that your body can easily react to with something your body isn't necessarily used to breaking down. Better the devil you know, than the devil you don't.

What also makes fat-free foods basically worthless is that your body actually needs some fat to burn fat. That's why there's a fat chance you'll get skinny, or stay skinny, without them. Fats provide double the energy of carbs and proteins, help you feel full, and are necessary in the absorption of many nutrients. By eliminating them from your diet, you're actually doing yourself a disservice. What you're saving in fat may not be worth what you are getting in unnecessary and unhealthy ingredients.

That doesn't give you carte blanche on fatty foods. You should always try to stick to unsaturated fats when possible. Reduced fat (25 percent less fat than normal), low fat (3 grams of fat or fewer), and "light" (50 percent less fat or one-third of the calories) are better choices than fat free, but you still have to be careful with these too. For example, reduced-fat peanut butter has only 10 fewer calories than regular peanut butter but has many more additives. Reduced-fat Oreos are another example, as they have only 1 gram of saturated fat (versus 2 grams in a regular Oreo), but they have approximately the same amount of carbs, sugars, and sodium.

Sugar-free products* won't get you anywhere—unless you were planning on running to the bathroom. These foods are normally filled with artificial sweeteners since something has to

---

* If you're diabetic, you should speak to a medical professional about what foods to eat and what substitutions to make in your diet to ensure it's proper, healthy, and balanced.

be added to make the foods taste good if natural sugar is taken out. These additives may inhibit weight loss, cause cramping, and lead to other things associated with stomach pain (we'll leave that to your imagination). Unless you are a diabetic, your body is used to digesting natural forms of sugar. Sugar free foods aren't necessarily lower in fat or calories, so make sure to read labels because you might be losing the taste for no good reason.

As you can see, there are high costs associated with these "free" products. That's why you should just try to stay away from all of them. If you want to have a diet lower in fat or refined sugar, lean toward foods that naturally don't have them, as opposed to those that need replacements. Unless you are under specific orders from a doctor in which you have to elim-inate certain food groups, a well-balanced diet of "real" foods is the ideal way to eat. By "real," we mean a diet rich in fruits, vegetables, whole grains, lean protein, low-fat dairy, and healthy unsaturated fats (like avocado, olive oil, nuts).

For those times when you're going to indulge in a treat, go for a smaller bite of the actual cookie, chip, or snack. Stay away from impostors such as sugar-free and fat-free foods. Just as those fake gold watches turn your wrist green, imagine what these foods are doing to your body!

23. Are protein bars a snack food, a meal replacement, or are they just glorified candy bars?

Just like some girls in high school, protein bars have become very popular because they're easy! However, that doesn't make them the cleanest or healthiest choices, nor does it mean that they are full of substance.

Most protein bars are heavily marketed as being healthy, but some of them are way worse for you than a Snickers. To ensure you're not getting a candy bar in disguise, look for a bar that has 15 or more grams of protein and 3 or more grams of fiber. The calories should range from 150 to 200 and no more than 5 grams of fat and 8 grams of sugar. When you're looking at the label to find this information, you must also look at the serving size. Make sure to do the math and multiply everything listed on the nutrition panel to know the true story of what's really in it. For example, some labels may say the serving size is two or that the serving size is half of the bar. This is really the same thing, and the amount should be doubled to know how much protein, fat, calories, sugar, and carbs you're really consuming.

When looking at the labels, also avoid bars with more than 5 grams of saturated fat and those that contain artificial sweeteners, palm oil (also may be listed as palm kernel oil), or soy protein isolate. Try to find one that is well balanced with 40 percent carbs, 30 percent protein, and 30 percent fat. While this may seem limiting, there are literally hundreds of bars to choose from to suit your wants and needs—crunchy, chewy, organic, gluten free, double protein, added fiber—and they all come in what sound like mouth-watering flavors. They can come in handy in a pinch when you're traveling, tight on time, or as an added pick-me-up before or after a workout. However, just because they are convenient, this doesn't mean you're going to get the same level of nutrients from a bar than you would from real food. So don't make a habit of using them as meal replacements or instead of fruits and veggies as a snack.

In the same vein that they're easy, you should also think of protein bars like a quickie—they can satisfy the urge, but most of the time you should want something a little more savory, satisfying, and lasting!

4. Should I eat before I work out?

Don't you hate it when your iPhone starts off with a full charge and then, despite barely using it, it's lost half of its battery life? This is the same thing that can happen to your body if you don't eat a little something before a workout. Even though you may wake up feeling full of energy, by the time you get your workout started, you may already feel drained if you haven't given yourself the proper fuel. Without it, you will probably get zapped of the energy you need to not only get your workout going, but also to keep up your stamina throughout.

If you work out in the mornings, we know it can be a real drag to have to get up even earlier to eat before a workout. However, to make sure it doesn't become a worthless workout, your body needs fuel to exercise. The only way it gets that is through calories, which you can only get from food. While having some nourishment is less important for low intensity workouts, if it's going to be mid to high intensity, then having a little something to eat beforehand can be very beneficial.

Stick with eating something small and choose easily digestible foods. You want to put gas in your tank, but too much or the wrong type might make you stall. Half to a whole banana, one or two slices of whole wheat toast or English muffin with nut butter, oatmeal, piece of fruit, handful of nuts, crackers with cheese, or hard-boiled eggs are all easy to prepare, delicious, and will help to put pep in your step. Combining protein and carbs are ideal, as they both work to increase your energy and support your muscles.

If you tend to work out later in the day or at night, try to time your exercise so you don't eat a big meal immediately beforehand. Get some distance between them so that you can go the distance without feeling weighed down.

If you like to work out to fight off your hangover, it's even more important not to work out on an empty stomach. The alcohol from the night before will likely impede your digestion. You'll have fewer nutrients in your tank as a result, and the workout could be a big-time struggle without food. While the last thing you may want to do is eat, it should help to give your body the extra nutritional *umph* that you're going to need to push through and sweat it out.

No matter how, when, or why you exercise, staying hydrated is just as important as eating. Water will help keep up your energy levels, cushion your joints, and help you not to huff and puff too much. Without it, you might cramp up, get dizzy or lightheaded, and lose focus. Keep a water bottle with you before, during, and after, and keep filling it up because you are losing water as you sweat.

Think of eating and drinking before you go out as an exercise aphrodisiac—it will get you up, keep you going, and make sure the heart is pumping.

25. Am I drowning all of my money in those fancy, enhanced waters?

The tides are turning. Plain water is now considered passé as new types of water are flooding the market.

Waters enhanced with vitamins were a refreshing change from the norm when they first emerged. The only problem was the word *vitamin*, since most tended to be low in them. Many of these waters are either missing or have less-than-optimal levels of essential vitamins and minerals. They also have way more sugar than nutrients. Did you know that you can get the same amount of sugar by eating approximately fifty jelly beans as you would get in one bottle of some vitamin waters? While there are some varieties that offer sugar-free options, they still may not offer the nutritional support you were hoping for. They can give you a false sense of security if you're using these drinks as a way to get your vitamins and minerals. Between the high sugar content and low levels of nutrients, not to mention the artificial additives, these vitamin waters are usually lacking in the healthy category. When you consider how much they cost, a daily multivitamin is a fraction of the price and you'll be getting way more for your money.

Other types of enhanced waters making a big splash are those that have electrolytes. Electrolytes (minerals including sodium, potassium, calcium, magnesium, phosphorous, and chloride) are very important for your body to function properly, as they help you stay balanced and hydrated. For those very active people or those who are dehydrated or sick, these types of waters or drinks can be beneficial. Be aware that some waters just have electrolytes added for flavor and won't do anything to replace your levels after a sweaty workout or when you're really sick. Be *smart!* Look at the labels and take note of the levels of the minerals designed to increase your electrolyte levels to see if you are really getting any benefits. While drinking any kind of water is a great way to stay hydrated, don't fool yourself into spending more money on these waters that don't have a lot of electrolytes in the hopes you're getting a lot of added value.

Coconut waters are trying to leverage the success of electrolyte waters since coconuts are a natural source of potassium. However, many only have one quarter of the potassium of a banana, while being eight times more expensive! Most also require you to drink a lot to get the hydration you're seeking. This will, unfortunately, come with a lot of sugar and empty calories, so they may be counterproductive.

There are also vitamin drops, flavor enhancers, and waters with a hint of fruit. There is even a new wave of really interesting waters that use artichokes, maples, watermelons, birch, and cactus. While these sound cool, just be careful of those that have outrageous claims or those with added sugar or artificial sweeteners and dyes. It might be better to try squeezing your favorite fruits into your water instead and avoid all the unnecessary sugar, empty calories, and unnatural ingredients.

While these designer waters are far from being washed up, there is nothing wrong with basic H_2O. If you don't like the taste of regular water, just dip one toe in at a time to make sure it's safe before you dive in.

6. I can't live without my soda, but what is it doing to my body?

We want to look like Beyoncé, Taylor Swift, and Sofia Vergara from their soda ads, too, but we have a feeling they aren't drinking too much soda since they still have those amazing bodies. Whether you prefer diet soda or regular soda, you should really try to avoid them both.

Regular soda has no nutritional value, so you're basically filling up a tall glass with sugar, calories, chemicals, and caffeine. While diet soda has less sugar and fewer calories, it tends to have more artificial sweeteners, additives, and chemicals that can deplete your body's calcium, do damage to your bones, teeth, and stomach, and have other negative health effects. Both types of soda have been reported to cause problems in the kidney and heart, and they can also lead to weight gain, obesity, and cavities. Sodas can also stain teeth and lead to signs of aging—both of which probably won't be reversed by all the teeth whitening and Botox you can afford!

Now that you know how bad it might be for you, do you think you'll be able to keep yourself from pouring another glass? Initially, probably not! That's because the sugars and sweeteners in soda can be addictive. These ingredients not only enhance the taste, but mess with your taste buds so you're always craving more. It's actually science that makes it hard to kick a soda habit, but don't let that leave you gulping for air!

The best replacement for soda is water. While it may not taste as good as soda at first, it will go down a lot easier if you remember it's calorie free, caffeine free, and sugar free! Ice cold water can be extremely refreshing, hydrating, and enjoyable. However, we know there are some who find water boring. If that's you, try adding a few slices of your favorite fruits (like apples, oranges, lemons, or strawberries) or combinations of them to your water. You can also get creative by adding cucumber or other flavor variations like mint, thyme, and ginger. If that's still not exciting enough for you, try unsweetened iced tea or natural hot tea. If it's the fizz you miss, try seltzers or other sparkling waters.

If you really can't live without soda, severely limit how much you drink because it really isn't a good choice for any generation!

27. **I have salads for lunch every day, and I'm still not losing weight. What am I doing wrong?**

There's nothing better than meeting your girlfriends to gossip and catch up over lunch—whether it's during the workday or, better yet, on the weekends. However, if you don't want it to turn into an intervention about your weight, it's important to remember that not only should you *not* have the same thing for lunch every day, but all salads are not healthy.

Eating the same thing frequently or every day is considered food jagging. Just like a child who gets stuck eating peanut butter and jelly or grilled cheese sandwiches for lunch every day, you are following the same pattern. Try to vary your lunches to help kickstart your metabolism by digesting different foods. In the same way it is important to change your exercise routine to challenge different muscles and keep yourself from getting bored, the same should be done with your meals.

Just because a meal has the word *salad* in it, it doesn't automatically make it a healthy or low-calorie choice. To figure out how your salad ranks, start by taking an inventory of what you've put in your bowl: what kinds of toppings, how much dressing, and how big is it? A good rule to follow when eating a salad is to stay away from iceberg lettuce, which has very few (if any) nutrients and fiber. Instead, use more nutritious greens, like kale, spinach, romaine, arugula, or mesclun. Fill your salad with unlimited veggies, but avoid peas and corn, as those tend to be starchy. Watch the extras such as cheese, nuts, seeds, crunchy things (like wontons, noodles, croutons, bacon bits) and dried fruits (raisins, craisins). Choose a lean protein, like grilled chicken, shrimp, turkey, tofu, eggs, or salmon, and avoid fried, breaded, and processed meats. Try to get dressings on the side and stick to two tablespoons or less. Avoid creamy dressings but know that light and fat-free dressings aren't necessarily a better choice. Even though they may be lower in fat and calories, they tend to be higher in sodium and sugar to make them taste better. Also, in order to absorb many of the nutrients in your salad, your body needs fats. Without them, you may not get the vitamins and minerals from the fruits and veggies you're eating. Kind of pointless!

If you tend to buy salads, be on the lookout, as some places put everything but the kitchen sink in a salad and drown in it dressing. They also tend to use really big bowls so you don't realize how much you're actually consuming. When it comes to salads, bigger isn't better and less is more.

28. What's the smartest way to cook my veggies?

Even if you're not an ace in the kitchen, you shouldn't be too intimidated to cook veggies. There are plenty of ways to prepare them, and even if some methods leave fewer nutrients than other ways, they're still vegetables and they're still healthy.

Traditionally, vegetables high in water-soluble vitamins (vitamins B and C) are the ones most sensitive to heat. If you want to cook these types of veggies, try to use a little bit of water and low heat for a limited amount of time. Carrots, spinach, asparagus, peas, broccoli, and zucchini are in this group.

On the other hand, vegetables that are higher in the fat-soluble vitamins (vitamins A, D, E, and K) do better when exposed to heat, so cooking them would be helpful in retaining these nutrients. Your body will also absorb these better if you combine them with some fat, so try cooking or topping them with a little bit of olive oil or butter. These veggies can include carrots, broccoli, spinach, tomatoes, and kale.

You might be noticing that some veggies fall in both categories. This is exactly the problem! It becomes a bit of a conundrum when you have vegetables in both camps. The same cooking method can both help and hurt the overall nutritional profile of whatever vegetable you're making. That's why you shouldn't concern yourself too much with how you're going to prepare them.

Other than frying and drowning your vegetables in butter or oil, there really is no bad way to cook your vegetables. While microwaving is a popular option for steaming, using an air fryer is also an easy and less time-consuming option where you can make the vegetables crispier and season to your liking. Whatever your preferred method, the more vegetables you eat, the better you'll feel and the more nutrients you'll get. While you may get fewer vitamins and antioxidants depending upon the method, it's hard to go wrong with veggies.

29. Fresh. Frozen. Canned. What's the difference when it comes to buying veggies?

Veggies have come a long way. Look at Brussels sprouts—from being the laughing stock when we were younger to now being on every trendy restaurant's menu. Vegetables are definitely making a comeback.

Ideally, you would have your own vegetable garden or live in an area that has access to good, fresh, and local farmers' markets. It's not always possible or probable to do this, which is why so many people buy their vegetables from conventional grocery stores.

While the vegetables in the store may look the same as those in a farmers' market, they actually could have many differences. Fresh vegetables in your basic supermarket are often picked before they are ripe, since they have to travel great distances to end up on your store shelves. In addition, they might have been exposed to light, heat, and less-than-optimal conditions. This might mean these vegetables may have fewer nutrients in them while having more additives and preservatives.

One way to combat this is to buy vegetables that are in season. This will increase your chances of getting the most nutrients and a better taste. You should also look for local signs. Many chains are now displaying that information. South America may sound exotic, but leave that for a vacation and not necessarily your produce.

If you find yourself in a pickle because it's close to impossible to eat in season and local all the time, don't forget about frozen and canned vegetables. Frozen veggies are a wonderful option because the freezing process occurs directly after picking and seals in all the nutrients. This way, even in the dead of winter, you can have peas, corn, broccoli, cauliflower, lima beans, and asparagus. Veggies from the freezer can also help you out because you can buy them ahead of time and store them without fear of them going bad. Don't go crazy with that, though; veggies don't go well with freezer burn! Besides, grocery stores tend to have sales on frozen veggies all the time, which makes them a great value. Stick with the steamed kind and lay off those in sauces, butters, and with lots of seasoning, as these can have high amounts of fat, sugars, sodium, and calories.

Canned veggies are also convenient and not just to use in your pantry as another shelf. They can be bought well in advance (and on sale) and stored for extended periods of time since they have long expiration dates. Make sure to wash them with water before you use or eat them, as this can help remove a lot of the extra sodium that's used to preserve them. Try to pick BPA-free cans or those in glass containers, if possible, to avoid the controversial chemicals.

When in doubt, buy whatever vegetable is available to you. Use the ones that are most cost-effective, fit into your routine, and that you think taste the best. Any veggie is better than none at all. So, no matter the season, you can eat and enjoy your favorite veggies.

30. I want to sizzle in the kitchen. What oil should I use and when?

Trying to figure out what type of oil to use and under which circumstances can put you on a slippery slope. Oil can be a wonderfully healthy option for cooking because it is low in saturated fat. Here are a few tips to keep in mind:

- **Usage:** Different kinds of oil have different temperatures at which they start to break down. This is known as their smoke point. Sunflower, grapeseed, avocado, canola, and refined safflower and sesame oils have a high smoke point, which means they can withstand a high heat. Therefore, these oils are great for sautéing, stir-frying, and baking. Oils like extra virgin olive oil have a low smoke point so they are much better suited for drizzling over cooked foods, salads, and breads. If you're unsure, and smoking occurs while cooking, stop what you're doing, throw it out, and start over. You don't want to use oil that's literally gone up in flames. Sometimes this can be avoided; some manufacturers list their recommendations for maximum temperature on the label. No matter what type of oil works for your meal, only use what you need, as the calories can add up.

- **Nutrient content:** Certain oils, like flaxseed and hemp, can be a source of omega-3 fatty acids. Since these nutrients can be affected by high heat, use these more for salad dressings. Other oils are high in mono-unsaturated fats, which can be good for the heart. These include avocado, olive, almond, and peanut oils.
- **Storage:** Most oils don't have a long shelf life. If your oil tastes or smells funny, you should probably throw it away. Flavor and scent are usually good indicators. To help them last, store in a cold and dark place. Also, the darker the bottle of oil, the better. This helps keep out the light that can negatively affect the oil.
- **Flavor:** If you're looking for something that won't change the taste, look for mild oils such as canola or vegetable oil. If you are looking to enhance the flavor, sesame oil, coconut oil, and nut oils can make a dish extra scrumptious.

- **Genetically engineered:** Many oils are sourced from genetically modified crops including soy, corn, canola, and cotton. If you're trying to avoid GMOs, you should probably avoid these varieties unless they are USDA Certified Organic or Non GMO Project Verified.
- **Purity:** Some extra virgin olive oils may be impostors filled with cheaper oil. How do you know you're getting the real thing? It can be hard to tell for certain unless you work in a lab, so we're pretty much out of luck. However, good rules to follow are to stick with those that come in dark bottles and have third party certification.

So, oil up but don't "burn, baby, burn."

31. **What's everyone's beef with eating burgers?**

Mmmm mmmm mmmm. When it comes to burgers, it's hard to not want to sink your teeth into one. Whether plain or with cheese, with special sauce or just lettuce, tomato, and pickles, they all sound so delicious. The most common burgers are those made from meat. Both lean ground beef and lean ground turkey breast burgers can actually be a great source of protein and contain essential nutrients, like selenium, niacin, B6, and zinc. While many people believe turkey burgers are healthier, that's not always the case, especially if you're not buying lean turkey meat. Regular ground turkey meat usually has both the skin and dark meat ground in. This can add a considerable amount of saturated fat and calories. Bison or venison burgers can be great alternatives, as they are juicy and savory while also being lower in fat and calories.

Fish burgers have been floating around on menus as well. They're not only lean, but high in omega-3 fatty acids and protein. However, don't have them too often because of high levels of mercury—skip the tuna burger and go for a salmon burger instead.

If you love to cook or grill, any of these varieties can be made at home. For meat burgers, try to buy lean ground meat or patties, and if you can find grass-fed, that's a bonus! Make sure to look at the ingredient panel and try to avoid purchasing those that have added seasonings or sauces and those high in sodium.

Veggie burgers have also become very popular, and not just on meatless Mondays. Whether they're pure vegetable, black bean, lentil, or chickpea, they tend to be higher in fiber, vitamins, and minerals than beef, turkey, or fish burgers. However, they also tend to be lower in protein. That is why so many of them use soy protein isolate to beef up the protein content. This holds true with many of the vegan and meat-alternative options. Try to avoid purchasing veggie or vegan burgers with soy protein isolate. To help you feel fuller and more satisfied, combine the healthier patties with non-processed cheese, hummus, or sliced avocado. Also, when buying these packaged in a store, make sure the first few ingredients are vegetables. Be wary of those that are highly processed with long lists of ingredients, high in sodium, or use various oils that are high in saturated fats. Beyond Burger and Impossible Burger come to mind, so check labels if you're just picking these options because you think they're healthier than a beef burger (and not because you're on a vegan diet). What's a veggie burger if there are hardly any veggies?

Generally, the worst part about having a burger is not the patty itself. It's all the stuff you pair with it that can be worse for you than the actual burger. Whether at home, at a restaurant, or even a fast-food joint, stick to a single patty. Cut out all the mayo, bacon, processed cheese, blue cheese, and fried onions that often come with your burger. A typical supermarket bun contains approximately 100–150 calories, so only cutting this out won't make a huge difference. This is great news for those of us who don't like eating a naked burger. However, if you're looking to eat low-carb or make small cuts that add up over the course of a day, you can always scoop it, switch to whole grain for some added fiber, or replace it with deli flats, English muffins, or lettuce. If you really want a side, like french fries, use self control and limit the amount you eat.

2. **I used to only eat white meat, but now I really like dark meat. Is it bad that I've ventured over to the dark side?**

The answer to this question isn't black or white. The difference between skinless white and dark meat is that the latter contains about 30 more calories per 3 ounce serving. This may seem pretty negligible, but how many people really eat only 3 ounces, which is the size of a deck of cards? If you eat the servings that you normally get at a restaurant or that you buy in the grocery store, it's usually at least double that amount. So, if you eat these larger portions frequently and throughout the year, white meat skinless chicken or turkey can help you save on calories and avoid putting weight on your own legs and thighs.

While white meat may seem healthier, this may not always be the case. That's because most people tend to add lots of seasoning and sauce to white meat because it tends to be drier. Trying to make white meat taste better and juicier (and more like dark meat) means you're adding slabs of calories and fat. This happens when you glob on the marinades, add lots of breading, fry it in a ton of oil, or even pair your meal with fatty sides. All of these things may enhance the taste, but they're counterproductive to keeping white meat a healthier option.

That's why it's time to see dark meat in a new light. Dark meat doesn't need all the extras to make it taste good, so, by the end of the meal, it may actually be the lower calorie option. Not only is dark meat more flavorsome, but it also contains more B vitamins, zinc, iron, and selenium. These nutrients can help with normal growth, wound healing, antioxidant protection, energy levels, and fertility.

So, getting to the meat of the question—the differences may depend on how you prepare your meat. Whether you're into legs or breasts, try to keep it as *au naturel* as possible! Always try to remove the extra fat before you cook it no matter what type you prefer. The healthiest preparation is to grill or bake the chicken or roast the turkey. Stay away from heavy sauces and instead use seasonings or low-sodium marinades. If you want to keep the skin on during cooking to add some flavor, remove it before you eat. Not only is the skin itself higher in fat and calories, but it also retains the marinades.

Hopefully now you've seen the light and know that you no longer need to pick sides since both dark and white meat have benefits.

33. Is sushi really as healthy as I want to believe it is?

With sushi, you must be careful so that you don't end up getting a raw deal! The most common misconception is thinking that no matter what you order, sushi is healthy. However, that is not the case. Sushi is the classic example that size does matter.

Sushi is deceptive because, while it seems you are exercising portion control, you actually end up eating a lot of rolls to fill you up. Your mind thinks that ordering only three rolls is appropriate, but, in reality, you're actually ordering eighteen to twenty-four pieces. Depending on the type of roll, this can add up to well over 1,000 calories since you are consuming a lot of rice per roll (approximately ⅓ to ½ cup of rice per roll). Additionally, sugar and salt are usually added when the rice is made. This can lead to increased calories, unnecessary sodium, and an abundance of empty carbs.

Despite how many rolls you order and how much rice you eat, you probably still end up hungry about an hour after the meal. Why? Mainly because the disproportionate ratio between carbs and protein (in this case rice to fish) will leave you unsatisfied. Another reason is that your body may be playing a trick on you. Soy sauces tend to be high in sodium; even the low sodium soy sauce still contains a hefty dose. So you may leave dinner feeling full, but your body may not have had enough to drink (and we're not talking sake bombs). This can make you very thirsty, so your body's desire for water may be masquerading as the need for more food.

There are more than enough options at a sushi restaurant that can be filling and healthy if you pay attention to how and what you order. Try starting with a salad (dressing on the side) and have some edamame *or* miso soup to help fill you up so you don't overeat during the meal. You can also start off the meal with an appetizer, like chicken yakitori or sashimi, but avoid tempura whenever possible. When ordering rolls, try to get hand rolls, as they tend to be lower in calories. Limit the number of crunchy rolls, tobiko, those with mayo and cream cheese (like a Philly roll), and the fancier rolls with lots of fish and toppings as these can all be high in saturated fat, cholesterol, and calories. No matter the roll, try to request brown rice whenever possible. Brown rice has more fiber (which will help fill you up and keep things moving) and it can help keep your blood sugar stable as well. Brown rice also contains magnesium, manganese, zinc, and vitamin E, while also having fewer calories. If you want to limit the rice, there's always sashimi, riceless sushi, or other entrées, like a teriyaki dish.

Ginger and wasabi are great ways to spice up your rolls. Not only will they help enhance the flavor, but they also have anti-inflammatory and immunity properties and can help fight bacteria and nausea. However, don't get confused between raw ginger and ginger dressing, as the dressing tends to be very high in calories.

While sushi can be a great source of omega-3 fatty acids, certain fish are high in mercury and this can be problematic. Too much mercury can be harmful to your brain, heart, kidneys, and other vital parts of your body. That's why it's best to avoid ordering too many rolls with tuna including yellowtail, yellow fin, bluefin, and ahi. Instead, try to stick with those lower in mercury like salmon, eel, crab, trout, octopus, and sea urchin.

Even though the sea may supply most of our sushi, don't forget that veggie rolls can be a great, healthy, and tasty choice too. Rolls full of cucumbers, spinach, asparagus, and even avocado are lower in calories while still containing important nutrients. They are also usually a lot cheaper than non-veggie rolls, so your bill will be a lot easier to digest!

34. Spill the beans. What are some ways to make sure I get enough protein and nutrients if I become a vegetarian?

From vegetarians to vegans, there has actually been a rise in the number of Americans who are going meat free (and even dairy free). Whether it's for ethical or health reasons, or just taste or texture aversions, leaning toward vegetables, fruits, and grains can be just as healthy. It's recently become even easier to follow this kind of diet, as there are so many options now available. No longer does being a vegetarian or vegan mean that you have to eat only beans and tofu or that you have to shop in some random and obscure health-food store for suitable products.

While there are now plenty of awesome choices for vegetarian meals and snacks, don't forget to make up for common nutritional deficits when eliminating some or all animal products:

- **Protein**: Some foods high in protein are soy products, tofu, edamame, tempeh, nuts, beans, lentils, and seitan. If you're not vegan, you can also incorporate yogurt, eggs, cheese, and milk as these can be a great source as well.
- **Iron**: Try lentils, soybeans, chickpeas, seaweed, and grains like quinoa and brown rice. Nuts and seeds high in iron include pumpkin seeds, sunflower seeds, pine nuts, and cashews. Iron-fortified foods like cereals, bars, and waffles are also worth checking out. Make sure to increase your intake of vitamin C, as well, as this will help your body absorb the iron. So, add lemons, oranges, kiwi, strawberries, tomatoes, tomato sauce, peppers, potatoes, cauliflowers, and Brussels sprouts to your meals as part of your dish, on the side, or as a topping (like iron-fortified cereal with strawberries). Broccoli and dark leafy green veggies, like kale and spinach, are super vegetarian foods because they contain both iron and vitamin C.
- **Vitamin B12**: Think of fortified foods like soy milk and breakfast cereals. Nutritional yeast has vitamin B12 and is very versatile since it can be sprinkled on foods like pasta,

salads, soup, or vegetables. If you're not a vegan, you can also get this nutrient from eggs and dairy.

- **Zinc:** Tofu, tempeh, lentils, nuts, and grains are high in zinc. Sesame seeds, pumpkin seeds, walnuts, pecans, almonds, cashews, macadamia, peanuts, and brazil nuts are also a great way to get this important nutrient into your diet. Don't forget beans too. If they have scared you away because you don't want to pass too much gas, try soaking dried beans overnight to reduce their gassy effects. Also, by rinsing off canned beans, you can reduce the sodium levels by almost half. You can indulge in some dark chocolate (or vegan dark chocolate) for zinc as well.

- **Calcium:** Tofu, beans, broccoli, kale, arugula, seaweed, oranges, and soy milk are great sources of this important nutrient. Sesame seeds and almonds are also high in calcium. If you're not vegan, milk, yogurt, and cheese are good sources of calcium.

- **Vitamin D:** Vitamin D is hard to get from food in general. It's even tougher if you don't eat dairy. Try mushrooms, and soy or nut milks fortified with vitamin D.

You can also always look to add supplements that contain these nutrients for added nutritional support.

I eat well, so what's the point in a multivitamin?

Unfortunately, you probably don't eat as well as you think—and that's normal. We are busy people with limited free time and tight budgets. It's hard to consistently make healthy choices all day, every day. While we all try to make the best choices when it comes to what we eat, it's not always possible or probable.

Add to that, when you do make healthy decisions, they may not be as nutritious as you think. For example, the USDA recently stated that it takes seven cups of today's spinach to equal the nutrition that a single cup provided in 1960. (Imagine what Popeye would look like now!) While spinach is still a good choice to include in your diet and will provide good amounts of vitamins and minerals, it's not what it used to be. The same thing is true with other fruits and vegetables. Many of our crops are grown in soil that may be depleted, over-farmed, or not fortified. This means people are often receiving less-than-optimal nutrients from the foods they eat. These facts don't eliminate the need to eat healthy, since you'll always get more nutrients from fruits and vegetables than you would from anything else. It does help prove the point as to why supplementing with a daily multivitamin is important, though.

Multivitamins, after all, are dietary supplements. This means they are meant to be taken in addition to, and not instead of, a healthy diet. Think of a multivitamin as your insurance policy for well-being. There's life insurance, car insurance, and health insurance—think of a good daily multi as your body's insurance . . . and the premium is much less! The average cost of most good multivitamins is less than a cup of coffee each day. It's a steal and a great deal!

For a good, comprehensive multivitamin, look for one that includes vitamins A, C, D, and E. Make sure the formula also has B vitamins and don't just look for those with numbers like B6 and B12. Thiamin, riboflavin, niacin, folic acid, biotin, and pantothenic acid are also B vitamins and are very important nutrients that should be included. Don't forget to make sure they include minerals like calcium and magnesium. Some brands will just say "multi" and you'll assume these minerals are in the product, but they aren't always there. Look at the supplement facts panel or make sure the label says multivitamin and mineral. Music notes are just sounds until they're strung together to make an amazing song. Vitamins and minerals act in the same way. Together, all these nutrients work in harmony to help support your body in many ways, including with stress and energy, metabolism, immunity, bone strength, and even healthy hair and skin.

Pricing of multivitamins can be misleading. To properly calculate how much a daily dose is, make sure to check the serving size and don't assume it's one per day. If you see a bottle of ninety vitamins for nine dollars, you would be psyched that it's a great deal—ten cents a day for three months. However, when you read the label and find out that it's actually three a day, you will only be getting a one-month supply for thirty cents a day. That is a big difference. Additionally, better vitamins aren't always more expensive and cheaper vitamins aren't always a better deal. It really depends on what is and isn't in the formula. Certain attributes like vegan, kosher, organic, and non-GMO ingredients may have premium pricing.

A good multivitamin and mineral does not give you the license to eat like crap and shouldn't be your only source of vitamins and minerals. The best way to assure you get what you need is to get as many nutrients as you can from a well-balanced diet, and use the multi to help make up for whatever your diet is still lacking. Good support is everything, as anyone who has ever worn a shoddy bra can tell you. How many people would say no to a natural lift?

Section 2:
The Inside Scoop on a Healthy Lifestyle

"I feel the same way about clothes as I do about food.
I want everything." —Mindy Kaling

36. **When I go out for dinner, what are the healthiest types of foods at the different types of restaurants?**

No longer do we need to travel to Epcot Center to get an out-of-this-world bite! Cities and towns throughout the country now have such an eclectic mix of restaurants that we're all able to enjoy many different cuisines.

If it's the taste of **Italian food** that you love, you know they get you right at the beginning. Be wary of the bread basket as the best is yet to come. For appetizers, stay away from fried foods—and that doesn't just mean calamari. Fried zucchini and eggplant are not any better. Just because it's made using vegetables doesn't mean it's any healthier. For dinner, lay off dishes with heavy cream sauce (a la vodka or alfredo) or lots of cheese (like raviolis and stuffed pastas). Instead, pick pastas with a marinara sauce and try to include veggies and/or protein in it. Tell your server you don't want the grated Parmesan cheese or make sure you know when to say "when." If you tend to eat your whole bowl of pasta, try ordering a hard to eat noodle (like spaghetti). It will take you a little bit longer to eat, so it will automatically slow you down and you should end up eating less because your body will have more time to know it's getting full. For chicken or meat dishes, pick entrées that aren't fried and stay away from those that come in layers with other cheeses, meats, and heavy sauces.

Asian fusion restaurants are hard to resist, too. If you are looking for an appetizer, wonton soup is a great choice, but egg-drop soup? Not so much. Dumplings can be a low-calorie option, steamed obviously more so than pan-fried, and veggie more so than pork. For main meals, most Asian restaurants offer a great and healthy assortment of vegetable, fish, seafood, meat, and chicken options. Many of these dishes are well-balanced since they incorporate veggies, protein, and carbs. However, it's the preparation that turns something healthy into something unhealthy. For instance, steamed chicken with broccoli with sauce on the side is a totally different meal than sesame chicken (i.e., fried), so pay close attention to the cooking methods, the type of sauce, and the amount of sauce. Also, be careful of the starchy sides. Even the little take-out containers of rice or noodles are deceiving because they actually hold a lot more food than you would think. Watch out for tofu dishes as well. Most restaurants fry or marinate it in a lot of sauce to get it to taste better, so it's not always healthier. As for sushi, keep portions in check, go for low-sodium soy sauce, and stay away from tempura rolls and those with lots of fish and toppings. (For more info on sushi—see page 58.)

Like Asian food, **Indian meals** also tend to be well-balanced, as they offer a ton of vegetables with protein. As an added bonus, Indian dishes tend to incorporate lots of beneficial spices like turmeric, ginger, and chiles. Lean toward roasted, steamed, or boiled meats that leave out the heavy sauces and extra calories sometimes associated with this type of cuisine. Look for tandoori options, such as chicken or shrimp, which can be leaner and lighter entrée choices. Stay away from those meals made with coconut milk, lots of oil, or ghee. Naan and basmati rice can be high in calories, so if you like having them, stick to a small serving of each.

Mediterranean/Greek food is a must-have, as well. To start, don't fill up on hummus and pita. Even though there are some health benefits associated with chick peas, there are so many more benefits from the food you're going to eat later on that's just as delicious. These foods tend to combine healthy fats with whole grains, which is a win-win. Stick with the grilled and seasoned fish or chicken that usually come with a hefty amount of veggies. If you love a Greek salad (and who doesn't), don't go overboard with the feta cheese and try to get the dressing on the side since most restaurants tend to use a very generous amount. Souvlaki can also be a great choice for an appetizer or a main meal, as it's a good combination of meat/shrimp/chicken and vegetables. Gyros can be high in calories, so only have them once in a while.

The **French** are famous for their food for a reason, but you have to be careful when ordering. Say au revoir to cream soups, béarnaise, béchamel, hollandaise, and beurre blanc sauces, which are all very high in fat and calories. Also bid adieu to au gratin dishes and melt-in-your-mouth baguettes. Where does that leave you? Still with plenty of delicious options! Enjoy entrées that are steamed, grilled, roasted, or poached and those in light wine sauces. Pick broth-based soups, chicken instead of duck, and if you can't resist the frites, get one order for the table to share. If French food isn't worth eating without your favorite sauce, get it on the side and use it sparingly.

Last but not least is **Mexican Food**, where you always feel like you just walked in to a fiesta! How can you not have a good time when the drinks are flowing and the food is hot hot hot? Be careful, though, as many restaurants tend to get you with the chips and dip as soon as you walk in the door. Guacamole and salsa aren't your enemies, but the chips can do you in. Take a handful and put them on a side plate so you can keep track of how many you have eaten and do not ask for another basket. These chips also tend to be very salty so make sure to drink a lot of water (and don't just turn to a margarita). Dehydration has a lot of the same symptoms as hunger, so this will help to ensure you don't overeat throughout the meal. As you order, try to avoid the dishes that have a lot of cheese and sour cream. Also try to stay away from fried shells, flour tortillas, fried burritos, refried beans, and rice. Instead, order ceviche or gazpacho to start and soft whole grain tortillas, lettuce wraps, fajitas with grilled veggies, or steamed fish for dinner. You can also check out the a la carte menu as there are usually healthier choices listed. Don't be afraid to use salsa, cilantro, lemon, and lime to add flavor and make the food muy bueno.

37. How much weight can I possibly gain following a bender weekend?

One person's bender weekend could be another person's regular Saturday or Sunday. So, for these purposes, it's important to distinguish what we define as a bender weekend. We're imagining a totally gluttonous time away (perhaps in Vegas)— where bottles are popping, food is flowing, and days roll into one another . . . but that may just be because we haven't gotten away in a while. With that said, it can also be a bachelorette party, a two-day concert, a sporting event, a holiday getaway, or even a staycation where the only objective is to have fun and indulge.

While the weekend may be hard to forget and even harder to remember, if you constantly eat and drink nonstop, the pounds could become an unwanted souvenir. One pound is equivalent to approximately 3,500 calories, which isn't that hard to reach if you're throwing back drink after drink and eating like it's your last meal. While you're away, you're also probably not exercising and not sleeping, which won't help matters. That's why it's possible to gain a couple of pounds—likely one to two pounds a day. The more you eat and drink, and the less you move, the more unflattering your bathing suit will be by the end of the weekend. No, it's not the hotel mirror—your clothes *are* getting a bit tighter!

That doesn't mean it's something to get crazy about as long as reenacting a scene from *The Hangover* is not a frequent occurrence. If you had fun, deal with it. Accept the consequences; they shouldn't be too long-lasting if you go back to eating normally, drinking in moderation, and getting back to the gym. You should be able to take off any weight you put on in a reasonable amount of time. Give your body a few days to adjust and avoid the scale. There's no need to panic and you don't have to go crazy with long and intense workouts. You also shouldn't skip meals or starve yourself. If you go from over indulging to malnourishment, you're only going to screw up your body and it's going to take longer to regulate and get that weight off.

Most importantly, don't let this derail or discourage you if you stopped following your healthy eating plan. Otherwise, you're going to continue on this downward spiral and the weight of one bad weekend will be nothing compared to what's to come. You had a slip up. You're human. It's okay to live a little and enjoy yourself. You should just get right back in the game.

38. **All of my friends have been buying cleanses lately. Should I do one, too?**

Your body already has its own cleaning service and does not need any extra support to get the job done. Doing a cleanse is just like cleaning up after a housekeeping service comes to your home—pointless and redundant. Your liver, kidneys, and digestive system work their magic daily to rid the body of toxins and oxidants. It's a dirty job, so let your body do it!

Cleanses can be expensive and devoid of nutrients. Since they count on no or low intake of food, they can be dangerous and leave you lightheaded, moody, malnourished, and unable to focus. Once you re-introduce real food back into your diet when the cleanse is over, it's very likely that you will put the weight back on. It's also a very big possibility that you will return to your normal (perhaps unhealthy) habits, and end up even heavier than where you started. So, rather than focus on a short-term solution, it's a better idea to try to make small, permanent changes that can make a world of a difference.

Since your body already has to deal with so many things that are unavoidable (like pollution, germs, and aging), modifying things you can control will enable your body to work more efficiently, therefore rendering a cleanse worthless. Try to:

- Cut out all artificial sweeteners
- Stay away from added salt and sugar
- Avoid drinking alcohol
- Eliminate fried and high-fat foods, processed snacks, sugary treats, and soda
- Include foods that are high in fiber
- Focus on fruits, vegetables, and lean protein
- Drink lots of water and/or green tea. Add lemons, if possible, to further help flush out toxins.

- Exercise a few times a week, even if that just means a brisk walk for at least 30 minutes or taking a minimum of 10,000 steps throughout the day

These changes should help you to stop feeling "icky" and will leave your body in the best state to clean itself thoroughly, frequently, and without outside interference. There should be no reason to do a cleanse—it will just make more of a mess!

39. **What is more important—the amount of calories or the type of calories you consume in a day?**

If two people were given 1,600 calories per day and one chose to eat fruits, vegetables, whole grains, and lean proteins while the other person ate foods full of refined sugar, fried meat, and fatty and processed snacks, would you consider these equal? Other than having the same amount of calories, it's hard to say they are similar in any other way.

That's why just counting calories won't always result in weight loss. Since calories are responsible for your body's energy, it's much more complex than just keeping count. You need to look at where they're coming from, in addition to how many you have. Take two women who both weigh 150 pounds. If you were going to try to figure out which one was in better shape, would you be able to answer this based on that number alone? Or, would you want to know their height, daily diet, exercise routine, genetics, and muscle tone? As our math teachers taught us long ago, numbers have meaning!

A good combination of calories from carbs, fats, and protein will help your body efficiently metabolize them. By sourcing your calories from foods high in vitamins, minerals, fiber, and other essential nutrients, your body will have the fuel it needs to get through the day and store only what is necessary. On the opposite spectrum, empty calories have no nutritious value so you're adding to your total count without getting any real benefit. It's like buying a shirt on final sale but realizing when you get home it's damaged. You got a great bargain, but you have nothing to show for it and you can't even use it or get your money back.

That doesn't mean that you shouldn't keep your calories in check. Too many can lead to weight gain. Too few are not always the answer either. An insufficient amount of calories will decrease your energy levels and leave you sluggish. You will also be less likely to be full and more likely to overeat later on.

You have to find that right balance, and eating healthy foods throughout the day will help you achieve it. Forget about focusing on only the total number of calories and remember, it's quality *and* quantity. Think of it like you do your age: as Abe Lincoln said, "In the end, it's not the years in your life that count. It's the life in your years."

Is watching what I eat more important than hitting the gym?

What you put in your body matters more than what you do with your body. It often takes less effort (albeit more willpower) to avoid a bag of chips than it does to find the time to make it to the gym. Both will save you the same amount of calories, but one involves a split second decision and the other at least a half hour out of your day.

Cutting calories doesn't mean you have to cut out food. By making smart choices, a little can go a very long way. If you were to replace processed snacks with fruits and vegetables, fried meats with lean proteins, and white flour with whole grains, you would be saving a heck of a lot of calories. Even just scooping your bagel would make a difference. By watching the quantity and quality of the calories, you'll be more likely to see the scale as your friend.

But watching what you eat shouldn't eliminate the importance of working out. Low- and high-impact workouts, along with lifting weights, will burn calories. By adding exercise to your weekly routine, you can also build muscle. Muscle helps to burn more fat, which, in turn, burns more calories. Exercise can also help you sleep better, reduce stress, and release powerful endorphins. Together, all of these will help you lose weight and be in a better mood. It doesn't give you a free pass to chow down. If you find the time for a heart-pumping workout, but don't change the way you eat, you may not reach the goals you set for yourself.

That's why it's best to combine working out with a healthy diet. The two really work hand in hand, and you can burn more calories doing these together than you would with just one or the other.

1. Will cutting out dairy help me moo-ve the scale in the right direction?

The slogan "Got Milk?" isn't just a cute ad campaign with good-looking famous people flaunting their milk mustaches. There is actually a reason your body wants and needs the nutrients that dairy products can provide. Dairy is rich in calcium, vitamin D, potassium, and protein. The body needs these nutrients to support strong bones and teeth, and they can even be helpful with preventing osteoporosis later in life. So, unless you want to take off a few pounds by losing teeth and breaking bones, it may not be the best idea to eliminate dairy in hopes of losing weight.

This doesn't mean that you should go crazy and become a Dairy Queen. Whole-fat dairy products tend to be high in saturated fat so, instead, try to stick to low-fat yogurt and milk. These can still give you the important nutrients without all the excess calories. If they don't fill you up, or you don't like the taste as much, stick with a small amount of the real thing. For example, a regular 5-ounce Greek yogurt can be a better choice than adding toppings and sweeteners to a non-fat variety just to make it taste better.

That's why it's so important to find the right balance of feeling full without overdoing it. After all, to drop a few pounds, it's all about total calories in and total calories out. It is not about removing an entire food group. Dairy products alone won't make you tip the scale. You just have to avoid the cartons of ice cream, the gallons of milk, and the blocks of cheese. It's eating *like* a cow and not *from* a cow that is probably making you feel that you need to lose a few pounds.

If you have an allergy or sensitivity to dairy, are vegan, or still feel the need to remove it from your diet, it's very important to make sure you incorporate other foods to ensure you are getting enough calcium, vitamin D, and potassium. Look for fortified foods or milks sourced from rice, nuts, coconut, hemp, or soy. Also try to add more tofu, beans, leafy greens, broccoli, nuts, and oranges into your diet. Supplements can also provide these nutrients as well.

42. Does it matter if I skip breakfast?

While most people would never leave the house without washing their face and brushing their teeth, they often have no problem skipping breakfast even though it's just as crucial. There is truth to what your mom said. Breakfast really is the most important meal of the day. Eating a good breakfast gives you the fuel your body and mind need to get going. Those who consistently eat breakfast are more likely to have a mental edge over those who don't. They also tend to be more focused, better able to concentrate, and have more energy and alertness. Those who skip breakfast are reportedly moodier and more sluggish, which probably makes them pretty unpleasant to be around.

Eating breakfast can also help turn your skinny dreams into a reality. By nourishing your body first thing in the a.m., you will most likely stay fuller throughout the day. With hunger pains at bay and food in your stomach, you should be better able to make healthy choices and keep up the good work. It may seem that by cutting out breakfast, you would be saving calories and therefore more prone to losing weight, but it actually can have the opposite effect. While it is true that you have to cut calories or burn calories to lose weight, depriving your body of important nutrients first thing in the morning can be counterproductive. As the day goes on, you will probably end up snacking more or overeating at other meals as you will be playing catch-up. This often results in more calories than if you just had a healthy breakfast when you first woke up.

Eliminating breakfast can mess with your metabolism, as well. The longer you delay eating, the slower your body will start to burn calories and expend energy. By not feeding your body within an hour or so of waking, in many ways you're hitting your body's snooze button and it will take longer for it to get to work.

If you incorporate breakfast each and every day, your body will respond. A hearty breakfast will supply you with the fuel and nutrients you need, and that is the best kind of wake-up call.

43. Will smoothies fast-track weight loss?

If you're looking to lose weight or watch your sugar intake, you may not want to go bananas drinking smoothies. Smoothies can be very high in calories. Just think about how much fruit you have to put in a smoothie compared with what you would put in a bowl to eat—you would end up with a monstrous fruit platter to match the fruit you put in your smoothie. Additionally, many people use juice, peanut butter, milk, yogurt, and other ingredients that consequently increase the amount of calories and sugar. This is why many smoothies can rack up 500 to 600 calories, which is almost as much as a Burger King Whopper, a small Dairy Queen Blizzard, two slices of pizza, two Dunkin' donuts, or a bagel with cream cheese. Just as you wouldn't consider any of these meals part of a healthy balanced diet, a smoothie isn't the healthiest choice either.

If you drink smoothies with a meal instead of as a meal replacement, then your calories are really going to add up.

If smoothies are convenient for you to grab on the go, or if you use them to get fruits or vegetables into you or your children's diets, there are a few ways to make it healthier. Use a total of 1 cup of fruit, throw in spinach, cauliflower, or kale for added bulk, and try to use water, skim milk, or plain Greek yogurt as the base. It's also better to make it yourself than to go store-bought. This can help keep the size down, the ingredients low, and the cost will be more manageable, too!

If you want to enjoy the fruits of your hard work in the gym and the kitchen, then smoothies may not be the answer you're looking for.

44. **Dessert is my favorite part of the day, but I don't want to look like a cream puff. What's the healthiest option?**

There are three things that are guaranteed in life: death, taxes, and the right to eat dessert. After all, life is sometimes better with desserts! Generally speaking, it's okay to treat yourself every day. There is no reason to deprive yourself as long as you keep it to a small sampling or few bites.

The healthiest options would be a bowl of fruit, frozen grapes, Greek yogurt with berries, or an apple with peanut butter. However, there are times when we know that won't cut it. On those nights, try to keep it to 150 calories, which is equivalent to two to three squares of dark chocolate, a couple of small cookies, or an individual chocolate pudding. You could also choose a few spoonfuls of ice cream or sorbet, a Yasso bar, a baked apple, a popsicle, or even a small brownie. The key here is *or* not *and*.

You don't have to worry so much about the fat and sugar content as long as you stick to just a little bit. This should be doable, since you're allowing yourself to have something when you need it, so there's no reason to go overboard. Knowing you can treat yourself to another few bites tomorrow, you shouldn't feel the need overdo it today.

If you prefer homemade desserts, there are some easy ways to give them a nutritional edge. One trick is using unsweetened apple sauce, prune purée, or canned pumpkin instead of butter or oil. This can help lower calories without interfering too much with texture or taste. Another tip is to use 100 percent whole wheat flour instead of white flour. This may make your dessert a bit heartier. If that won't fly, try using a combination of half whole wheat and half regular flour, which should help keep the original consistency.

While it may be easy to behave well at home, it can be hard to use restraint at restaurants. They tend to believe when it comes to portions, the bigger the better. When the dessert tray crammed with oversized molten chocolate cakes, tempting pastries, and assorted pies is staring you in the face, it's almost impossible to resist. The berry bowl just doesn't compare. When ordering, try to avoid desserts with heavy cream, lots of whipped cream, ice cream, syrups, and toppings. Restaurant desserts are decadent enough; you don't need to choose one with all the extra accoutrements. Also, try to pick a dessert that the whole table will enjoy. With lots of spoons or forks, everyone can share—forced portion control!

No matter where your dessert comes from, make sure you're having it as a sweet treat, and not because you're still hungry after dinner. If that's the case, eat healthier foods that have fiber, protein, and nutrients so you can feel full and you won't be looking to your dessert to fill you up. Once you're satisfied, *then* you can go for the small treat as a night delight.

As long as you keep the portion size small, a moment on the lips won't last a lifetime on the hips.

45. Is salt the next four-letter word?

Your body needs salt to work. Your cells need it to function properly and, since you can't make it yourself, you need to get it from food. Without salt, our muscles, brain, heart, hormones, balance, and equilibrium would all be negatively affected. Your body also needs salt after you sweat, so whether you're active at the gym or just a hot mess, chances are you're going to need to replenish it daily. Trying to avoid salt completely can be bad for your health.

It's also basically an impossibility. Salt is in frozen, packaged, processed, and store-bought foods. Even though it is found in almost everything we eat, don't freak out. While many guidelines recommend that we should have ½ teaspoon to 1 teaspoon per day, the amount you consume is probably still within that range. If you have cereal for breakfast, a turkey sandwich for lunch, chicken teriyaki with rice and frozen vegetables for dinner, a handful of pretzels and a Greek yogurt for snacks, you're still below 2,000 milligrams of sodium for the day, which is less than 1 teaspoon of salt.

Unless you have high blood pressure or another medical condition in which your doctor told you to limit salt, your body can normally handle this amount and knows how to make the most of what it's ingesting. You can still add it (sparingly) to popcorn, pasta, and vegetables, or to enhance the taste of any of your favorite dishes. The tiny amounts you use in each of these instances are nothing to be concerned with.

If you tend to be thirsty constantly, swollen, or have high blood pressure or a serious weight issue, it is a good idea for you to speak to a doctor about limiting your salt intake. If they recommend cutting back or if you feel that you consume a lot of sodium, limit processed and packaged foods. Beware, though: salt is a master flavor masker and foods with lower sodium may not taste as good to you.

When it comes to sodium, watch your intake but take all the chatter with a grain of salt!

46. **I'm trying to watch what I'm eating, but it would be a buzzkill if I had to cut out all alcohol. What's my best option?**

If you're following a strict diet, not only do you deserve a drink, but you could also probably use one! Keep it to casual drinks and don't turn it into a boozefest. Too many drinks will not only add lots of calories, but they can impact your judgment, causing you to potentially drink more than you set out to in the first place.

Alcohol has no nutritional value; therefore, it contains empty calories. Try as you might to justify the piña colada by telling yourself that coconut has some nutritional benefits, it just doesn't work that way. The average 6 oz. glass of white or red wine will set you back around 150 calories while the same size piña colada clocks in at around 450 calories! That's 300 more calories with no nutritional benefits whatsoever. So, instead of worrying about being called a lightweight, be a lightweight and make smart decisions when you're belly up to the bar. While you don't have to eliminate alcohol, try to keep it to no more than four to six drinks per week if you're trying to keep your weight down.

If beer is your drink of choice, stick with ultra low-carb beer, which has less than half the calories of regular beer. Be careful not to super-size your brew or have too many bottles, or you'll wish you were looking through beer goggles the next time you step on the scale!

If mixed drinks are your fave, think of these in the same fashion as your outfit before you go out at night: one accessory is all you need. Stick to one mixer and use club soda or sparkling water and try adding lemon or lime. If you miss your usual mixers, try just adding a splash. Also, try to avoid sweet and fancy cocktails like those that have sugar on the rim or those that come with little umbrellas. They may look pretty and taste great, but they're full of empty and unnecessary calories. If dessert cocktails are your thing (like a grasshopper, mudslide, or chocolate martini), you're out of luck. These drinks are indulgences and not necessary if you're watching your weight. Even though they may be liquid calories, they'll leave you both wasted and "waist-ed."

If wine is your go-to drink, make sure to have a glass and not a bottle. If straight drinks are what you prefer, you have our respect! It's important to remember that, ounce for ounce, the stronger the alcohol content, the heftier the calorie count, so just be mindful of how much you down.

And let's not forget: friends don't let friends drive drunk, so pick a designated driver, call a cab, or get an Uber. This ensures your night out won't be anyone's last call.

47. **I'm seeing all these products in the grocery store made from vegetables and fruits. Are they really better for you than the real deal?**

Walking down any aisle in the supermarket, you're sure to see cauliflower pizza, hearts of palm noodles, lentil potato chips, and broccoli rice. Companies are incorporating vegetables in many popular types of foods—but are they good for you or just good marketing? The answer isn't the same for everything.

Broccoli or cauliflower rice are usually just the pure veggie, which make them a good substitute if you're looking to cut back on carbs and increase your daily servings of vegetables. Hearts of palm noodles and rice, zucchini noodles (zoodles), spaghetti squash noodles, green pea snack crisps, and *That's It.* Bars are also examples of foods that serve as healthy alternatives to the original.

On the other hand, certain foods that use vegetables or fruits as the "base" need a closer look. Products that use cauliflower are currently taking over the shelves. You can find pizza, pasta, gnocchi, fried rice, chips, pretzels, taco shells, and mac and cheese. There are also now several options for snacks and cereals that use lentils, carrots, sweet potatoes, spinach, bananas, and strawberries. For all of these types of products, make sure to look at carbs, sugars, sodium, and fibers to ensure you're getting the benefits of using vegetables or fruit substitutes—you should be getting actual nutrition and not a lot of stuff that's just making it taste better. For example, sometimes a cauliflower pizza or pasta might have as many carbs as regular pizza or pasta, so you're not gaining any benefit unless you truly prefer the taste. So if you're looking to lose weight or eat healthier, remember that just because a vegetable or fruit is in the name doesn't mean it's going to be beneficial for you. Cali'Flour Foods and Palmini Pasta are good examples of healthier options, as they are made of pure cauliflower and pure hearts of palm. However, several other brands are not pure vegetable and instead combine the vegetable with added starches. That's why it's so important to read labels (specifically carb content for those on low-carb diets) to understand what exactly is and isn't in your food.

Bottom line: Many of these companies are trying to dangle the carrot in front of you as you walk down the aisle to make their vegetable-based foods appear healthier—but don't always assume that's the case.

48. Why is tea considered healthy?

Since tea is one thing in the kitchen that's hard to screw up (just add hot water!), it should be a relief to know it's good for you.

Of all the drinks out there, tea is probably one of the best. It doesn't matter if it's iced or hot, as both varieties can be healthy. Tea contains phytochemicals, polyphenols (which include flavonoids), as well as antioxidants. Tea can aid in digestion, immunity, boost your metabolism, support your bones, and help with stress and mood. Teas are also calorie free as long as you don't add anything to them like sugar, milk, or honey.

If you're looking to cut back on caffeine but not cut it out, tea can be a great alternative to coffee. Green, white, black, and oolong teas contain caffeine, while herbal teas do not. If you're confused, just look at the ingredients. If it lists tea, then you'll know there is caffeine. If it doesn't, there is none. That's because herbal tea is actually made from spices, dried herbs, flowers, and/or fruits and not tea leaves. Always read the labels though, especially when dealing with blends.

However, like all else, there are a few things you should know about drinking tea that we think might even surprise the queen!

- Don't drink tea while it's piping hot. Let it cool down a bit (but still make sure it's warm), because anything searing can cause problems in the stomach and digestive tracks.
- Don't over-steep your tea bags as it will probably get a nasty, bitter taste. Try to use loose leaf teas; they are often less processed (thereby containing more antioxidants).
- Try not to drink tea on an empty stomach, especially the caffeinated varieties. Bloating, dizziness, and other "drunklike" symptoms have been reported when the only thing in the stomach is the tea.

While it is possible to have too much tea, it is not likely. The media profiled one woman who reported negative effects to her health from tea, but she had more than one hundred cups of tea a day! More than one hundred of anything a day is usually not a good idea (unless it's exercise like sit-ups, push-ups, or jumping jacks), and who even has the time in their day to brew, drink, and make it the bathroom to pee out one hundred cups of tea?

For the rest of us, a few tea cups a day can be beneficial to our health and nothing to worry about. So sip it, enjoy it, and pinkies up!

49. For the sake of those around me, I need coffee! How many cups a day are okay to drink?

Your head hurts, you're groggy and foggy, and you can hardly function. It's not due to a late night out or because you're coming down with something; it's because you haven't had your first cup of coffee yet and haven't injected yourself with java.

Coffee has really become the acceptable drug of choice for so many. People often become addicted and turn into different, and better, versions of themselves after their initial cup of joe. They get jolted back to life and end up more alert and focused. While the caffeine acts as a mood enhancer, it isn't the only thing that makes coffee beneficial.

Coffee is a great source of antioxidants, can increase energy, and helps stabilize our moods. It can also help keep our brains healthier and our minds sharper. Coffee has been reported to help reduce the risk of heart disease and type 2 diabetes and can help with pain. Some studies have shown that it can help protect the skin against sun damage (but that doesn't mean you should throw away your sunscreen). There are also those who swear they can't "really" go to the bathroom without it; you can usually spot these people running to the nearest restroom with a look of sheer determination on their faces.

However, some people use coffee as a diuretic or to curb their appetite. This can be problematic and a bad habit to get in to. Others depend on it for their energy, which could be masking a bigger problem. If this sounds like you, it's really important to figure out why you're so sluggish without coffee. You should definitely make sure there's no underlying problem.

The other issue with coffee is the caffeine. Too much caffeine can potentially have negative effects. It can prevent or interrupt a good night's sleep and make us jittery or irritable. Caffeine is also extremely addictive. Since caffeine only stays in your body temporarily, you're constantly craving more and your body becomes dependent on it. Even decaf varieties usually contain some level of caffeine, so you're not necessarily out of the woods.

Three to five cups of coffee seems to be the magic number for how much coffee you can have in a day. While this is manageable, it doesn't mean it's necessary. Try to stick to one to two cups a day and be consistent with how much you drink and when you drink it to avoid crashing, headaches, or withdrawal symptoms. To avoid empty and extra calories and fat, avoid flavored shots or syrups and go for low-fat milk whenever possible. Stay away from whipped cream and added sugar or sweeteners (sprinkle cinnamon as an alternative).

So, coffee lovers unite. You don't need to give up your cup of java—and not just because we don't want to be in the cross-hairs when you stop. Whether you brew your own, or you get your daily fix from Starbucks (where your name may or may not be spelled correctly on your cup), as long as you keep your coffee habit in check, you'll avoid a latte problems.

50. Do I really need to drink eight glasses of water every day?

Just like it's hard to ever have too many shoes, it's hard to ever have too much water! The majority of our body weight is made of water and our systems are dependent on it. Water helps with regulation, digestion, hydration, metabolism, and immunity—and that's just scraping the surface. However, all day, every day, we are losing water. Just by breathing, peeing, pooping, and sweating, water is wasted. So, it's extremely important to replace it.

That's why you need to make sure you're getting enough of it. Eight glasses of 8 ounces of water per day, while not exact, is a good general goal. While that may seem like a lot, lucky for you, water is free and zero calories. Age, weight, health, diet, exercise routines, and geography help to determine if you need more than the 8 glasses. The heavier you are, the more water you probably need. If you live in a hot and humid climate (as evidenced by your hair constantly frizzing), chances are you need to increase your water intake. When you're sick with diarrhea or vomiting, you'll want to make sure you stay extra hydrated and always have a glass of water next to you to drink. If you're a gym rat, you'll need to have more water than someone whose daily exercise is walking from the kitchen to the couch. You can see just how many factors play into how much water you need.

If you don't like water or can't stand drinking it through-out the day, you're not out of luck. Fruits, vegetables, soups, teas, juices, and milk all count as being sources of hydration. Granted, they don't have as much water as good ol' H_2O, but they can help add to your total intake for the day.

The key to ensuring you're getting enough water is to stay ahead of it. Once you're thirsty, your body is telling you that you're a little late in the game. One way to gauge it is to follow the yellow brick road. If your pee is murky, try to get more fluids. If it's clearish, you're probably doing a good job staying hydrated.

While it is possible to drink too much water, more times than not, most people aren't drinking enough. So, don't worry about flooding your insides; you need plenty of water to keep yourself afloat.

51. **Does writing down everything you eat/drink really help with weight loss?**

Absolutely! Don't underestimate the power of a food log. We know sometimes it can be tedious and, quite frankly, a pain in the ass, but it really does help. In 2008, The Kaiser Center for Health Research in Portland, Oregon, did a study on weight loss comparing those who used a food diary and those who didn't. The people who recorded their food intake lost twice as much as those who did not keep track of their food. So, why does the simple act of writing this down help you lose weight?

You tend to be more mindful of what you are eating when you are held accountable. Whether you're writing it down, sharing it with a friend, talking to a nutritionist, or using a food journal app, keeping track of what you eat can help keep you in check. It will make you more aware of your choices and will usually cause you to think twice before making an unhealthy decision. Most people will cut down their calories and be smarter about what they eat when they see it written, and dropping pounds will usually follow. If you have an urge to eat junk (chips, candy, cookies, etc.) but know you have to write it down or that other people will see it (like a Registered Dietitian), you are more likely to skip it or to have a smaller portion.

This is why keeping an accurate food journal can help you lose weight. That is, if you're being honest. You have to lift up the curtain and put it all out there. The same way your hair colorist knows how gray you really are, and your bikini waxer knows how long it's been since your last appointment, there's no hiding from the truth. Sometimes, the only way to get results is to bare it all and be totally honest and upfront. To be as accurate as possible, write everything down as you go. If you wait until the end of the day, you are more likely to miss the "little" things, which add up. Don't forget to note your portion sizes.

A detailed log may help you realize if the size of your meals or snacks are out of whack and may need to be scaled down. Also, don't be afraid to admit to everything. If you have what you consider a bad day, don't leave it out! Admitting your mishaps will help ensure you are less likely to do it again.

Keeping track of what you eat can help you pinpoint what may be preventing you from reaching your goal weight. Analyze your daily entries at the end of each day. Take some time to look at what you ate and what you might be lacking. You may realize you are not getting enough fruits or vegetables, but have too many carbs. Recording your food is one thing, reviewing it and putting what you are learning into practice is another.

You can use a notebook, your phone, or even classic diary sheets to journal. Be sure to carry them with you at all times. There are also plenty of apps available for you to try. Just make sure you understand that it's not a perfect science. These apps don't always take your sex, height, and weight into account. They also don't necessarily have the perfect match for what you ate. This could over- or underestimate your caloric intake, so know it may not be precise. If you use them to gain a better understanding of what you're eating and how much you're eating, it can be very helpful.

No matter the type of journal you pick, remember you are the only part that really matters. The information you track is only as good as what you own up to, so you can't fool yourself any longer.

An Extra Scoop!

If you tend to be, or think you might be, an emotional eater, a food log can be extremely insightful and helpful. Life and emotions can be a huge part of what you eat and when you eat it. It's important to take note and write it down if you have certain feelings that send you to the freezer for ice cream. Keeping a food log can help you identify these triggers, as can speaking to a registered dietitian, therapist, or physician.

52. **In the supermarket, there are so many choices for snacks. What are the best ones when you've got the munchies?**

The perimeters of the supermarket usually hold the healthiest items like fruits, veggies, meats, and dairy. However, the middle aisles are where the party's at. As soon as you walk into this abyss, you can practically hear the sound of the snack bags opening. The lip smacking, drool-worthy, and mouth-watering reaction that follows is par for the course. As you're flirting with the idea of which ones to choose, there's often an internal dialogue on which snacks will help you avoid the walk of shame to the cash register.

The most important thing is not to get seduced by provocative words. Just because it says *smart, healthy, fit, thin, skinny, nature, natural* or *from the earth* doesn't mean it is any of those things. It might be, but it might not be. So don't automatically believe it's a good choice or a better choice—especially since you know what happens when you assume. Make sure to look at the nutrition facts panel to check it out for yourself. While these snacks might be lower in fat, they may still be more than you might expect, and even though they might use a few healthy ingredients, they might be amongst many unhealthy ones.

Reduced fat, light, popped, and baked snacks can be tricky as well. Although they have less fat than the originals, they may not have less sugar, sodium, carbs, or calories. Many times, they actually have more of these things or the differences can be nil. For example, Chips Ahoy regular chocolate chip cookies and their reduced-fat counterparts have a difference of 2 grams of fat. Other than that, their stats are pretty even, so there's not that big a difference between them. On the other hand, Nilla Wafers Original and the reduced-fat version have a much larger disparity between them, as the latter has significantly less of everything, so the reduced-fat variety is a healthier purchase. It really is a case-by-case basis.

While you might need to be Sherlock Holmes to get to the bottom of the reduced-fat case, you probably think that picking whole grain or multigrain over regular snacks would be an obvious choice. They are definitely healthier, right? Not always. In the case of Tostitos, the multigrain chips have 150 calories and 7 grams of fat for 8 chips while the originals have 140 calories and 7 grams of fat for 7 chips. These are more like twin products than sisters. Pretzels can be just as twisted. Snyder's Honey Wheat Braided Twists have more fat, sugar, and the same number of calories as the regular rods.

Confusing? In the words of Sarah Palin, "you betcha." That's why it's so important not to judge a book by its cover. You have to read all of the information and not just the headlines to get the whole story.

Once you can distinguish between the perception and the reality, if there is an obvious difference between snacks, pick the healthier one. There are some "better for you" versions out there, but you have to look carefully to find them. Look at the first few ingredients and the nutrition facts panel. Try to leave the snacks that have a ton of fat, calories, sugars, and sodium and those that use artificial sweeteners, partially hydrogenated oils, high-fructose corn syrup, and food colorings on the store shelf. That may not leave you with a lot of choices. These are all packaged snacks, so it's hard to find ones that are truly good for you. With that said, we know giving up your favorite munchies isn't a piece of cake. Just try to keep the junk out of the food or the junk in your trunk will take over.

53. **I can't keep up. Am I supposed to be counting grams of carbs or grams of fat?**

If it was as simple as cutting out fat or carbs, we would all know what to do to lose weight. With so many diet books and programs on the market, it's pretty obvious that this is a complicated question without an easy answer. There's a reason why the diet industry is such a big business. It has to cast a wide net, as what works best for one person may be totally different for another.

Generally speaking, there really is no difference between counting grams of carbs and grams of fat as long as you keep your calories in check. However, for you personally, there may be a huge difference. To properly figure this out for yourself, you first have to decide if you're more likely to restrict *how much* you're eating or *the types* of food you're eating. For example, if you love your carbs, you shouldn't have to give them up. Switch to whole grain versions instead of refined carbs and eat them with lean proteins, healthy fats, and foods naturally high in fiber. As long as you're watching your portions carefully, you should be able to keep your calories, fat, and sugar counts in check.

If you have no problem giving up refined and starchy carbs in your diet, then this may be the "weigh" to drop some pounds. That doesn't mean all fats and proteins are acceptable. Stick to lean meats, unsaturated fats, and don't use this as an excuse to load up on bacon, butter, and red meat. While you will be eating fewer carbs, it's still important to eat *some*. So, don't cut out all fruits, whole grains, legumes, and non-starchy vegetables.

In either case, it's about following a plan that you can stick with and that works with your lifestyle and schedule. Success is about losing weight gradually and keeping it off permanently.

We wish we had a foolproof answer that worked for everyone. Unfortunately for our bank accounts, we don't. What we do know is that the only way to lose weight is to take in fewer calories than you exert. Whether that's counting fat or carbs, only you know your path to least resistance.

54. **Can I still eat healthy if I am constantly eating out?**

Having someone cook your meal, serve the food, and clean up after you're done eating is definitely a luxury. But it can come with a hefty bill if you're not careful about what you eat—and we're not referring to just the check. At home, you probably have something small to start then a normally portioned main meal that may or may not be followed by a small treat. When you're out with friends and family, though, it's bread from the bread basket, Caesar salads and stuffed mushrooms, and an over-sized main meal. Add to that dessert and alcohol and you've probably consumed more calories in that one sitting than you would in an entire day at home.

That doesn't mean that you can't or shouldn't eat out. That would not only be unrealistic, but also who wants to live in a world where you can't dine out! There are ways to have your cake and eat it too!

- **Avoid these nine words/phrases**: creamy, fried, breaded, crispy, cheesy, drenched, slathered, all-you-can-eat, and unlimited. Instead, look for these four: grilled, broiled, baked, or steamed. Some restaurants mark their lighter and healthier options with a star or have them on a special part of the menu, so consider those too.

- **Sharing is caring:** If there are many items on the menu that look good, split them. Don't order them all. Pick your top choices and see if anyone else at the table will share them with you. If not, narrow it down to two options and get them both in appetizer portions. When it comes to dessert, apply the same philosophy. Get one or two to share, depending on the number of people with you, and ask for a lot of forks or spoons so everyone gets a few bites.

- **Mean what you say and say what you mean**: If you want to change the way something is prepared, just politely ask the server. Whether it's about swapping fried for grilled, putting the dressing on the side, eliminating an ingredient, or getting a main course as your appetizer, most chefs want you to enjoy the meal as much as possible and will accommodate your request if they can. If not, the worst that happens is the waiter will say it's not possible. If that's the case, then you can either choose another dish or have it the way it was offered. The days of being afraid of a waiter spitting in your meals are pretty much over—no restaurant wants to end up on Yelp or trending on Twitter with their own negative hashtag.

- **Don't drink anyone under the table:** It's always fun to have a cocktail (or two) or to share a bottle of wine at dinner. Sometimes, it even feels necessary when out with some family members. Try not to get too sloshed! The calories add up with too many drinks, and getting drunk tends to lower your inhibitions while increasing the likelihood you're going to make unhealthy decisions.

- **One size doesn't fit all:** Be mindful of portions. Restaurants tend to fill the plates and give us way more food than we need or want. Don't feel the need to finish it all at one seating. Yes, people are starving and it's not good to waste food. However, that's why leftovers were invented. Ask for a to-go bag and take it back home with you. Besides, how psyched will you be tomorrow when you open the fridge and realize you get to enjoy this awesome dish all over again and won't have to prepare lunch or dinner?

- **Take breaks:** It's really important to take some time in between bites. Whether it's to drink some water or just take a breath, this will help your brain catch up with your stomach and alert you when you're full. Also, halfway through your meal, take a five- to ten-minute break, especially if you eat quickly. By putting the fork down, you may realize you were just eating to eat and you didn't really need to wipe your plate clean. Make sure you only go back to eating if you're still hungry and need to finish your meal.

- **Make a game plan:** Check the menu before you leave home and go in with a strategy. Try to do this while you're not so hungry. If you know at which point during the meal you'll give yourself a treat, then you know the other times throughout the meal you have to make healthier decisions. Also, make a conscious effort to eat a little something before you go out. You don't want to go to the restaurant starving because, if it takes a while to order and for the food to come, you're probably going to inhale the bread basket and eat way too much.

Finally, get dressed up and enjoy it! The better and more attractive you feel, the more likely you will want to feel the same way when you leave the restaurant. It's never a good feeling to have to walk out with your pants unbuttoned!

55. **Are there foods that can help speed up my metabolism?**

Some of us are not as lucky as our friends who can eat whatever they want and not gain a pound. Most of us just look at food and put on weight. There is hope, though. Certain foods and behaviors can help boost our metabolism so all is not lost.

Start by eating breakfast within sixty to ninety minutes of waking to get things started. You have to use it or lose it—your body is in a state of fasting and you have to kick it back into gear. After that, make sure to eat well-balanced meals every three to four hours throughout the day. You have to eat frequently enough to keep things going at a good speed. If you slow down or skip meals, your metabolism will start to get a bit sluggish.

To give yourself a bigger boost, increase your intake of:

- *Protein:* Your body uses more calories to burn protein. Eggs, chicken, and fish are great sources and will help get your metabolism revved up.

- **Iron**: Low iron in your body can lead to a lower and slower metabolism. Think lentils, nuts, beans, red meat, spinach/leafy greens, Brussels sprouts, dark chocolate, and sunflower seeds. Don't forget about dairy and other sources of calcium, as these can also be helpful.

- **Capsaicin:** Just because you may not be able to pronounce it doesn't mean it's something you should avoid. Found mostly in hot peppers, like chili peppers, this spice can help give your metabolism a spark. You can eat these peppers raw or cook with them to heat things up!

- **Water:** Make sure to get in your eight glasses of water per day. If you're dehydrated, your metabolism will slow down. Some say that cold water is more helpful for your metabolism as it helps to burn a few extra calories. Normally, this would be insignificant, but if you're drinking eight glasses a day, those calories can add up over the course of a year. Some of us need all the help we can get.

- **Coffee and Green Tea:** Coffee can be helpful since it's high in caffeine and has been shown to help with focus, energy, and endurance—a triple threat. Green tea, which also contains caffeine but has catechins and EGCGs as well, has also been widely discussed as being a great catalyst.

While it all may start with your diet, it doesn't end there. It's vital to move and get off your hiney. Incorporate physical activity into your days and combine aerobic and strength training exercises into your weekly workout routines. Sleep at night is incredibly important, even more so if it's deep and restful.

It's also essential to avoid things that may be detrimental to your metabolism. This includes energy drinks. Even though they have a ton of caffeine, they also usually have many other ingredients (like sugars and artificial sweeteners) that could have negative effects on your body, including on your metabolism. That's the same reason to stay away from overly processed and packaged foods. Your body spends so much time trying to figure out what to do with these things that, in essence, other important processes get halted. Fatty foods, refined carbs, and even stress can also do the same thing.

While you may not naturally have a fast metabolism, it's still possible to get your motor running. By following some of these tips, you should be off to the races!

56. **What can I do to lose a few pounds so I can fit into my outfit this weekend?**

Don't you love it when you have the perfect outfit for a night out? You can see it in your head and picture how fabulous you're going to look in it. Then, unfortunately, reality settles in when you try it on and it just doesn't look like you remember. Such a deflating feeling! While jumping on the bed and breaking into a hardcore sweat while trying to get your pants to close could burn a few calories, there are some other ways that might work a bit better!

To lose one pound in a week, you have to consume approximately 3,500 fewer calories than you burn. A great way to do this is to eliminate about 500 calories per day. That may seem like a lot, but it's easier than you think and not so drastic. By reducing your caloric intake by 250 calories per day and increasing your exercise routine to burn an extra 250 calories per day, you'll have achieved the right balance.

To cut calories, start by swapping snacks. Forget the pretzels and chips and go for healthier alternatives like carrots, celery, cucumbers, or peppers. These can help satisfy your need for a crunch while making a dent in the calories you need to save. If plain veggies won't cut it, have them with a little bit of hummus or dip.

Next, eliminate processed foods—they're not natural and your body often doesn't know how to digest them. They also tend to have tons of sugar and/or fat, which won't do your figure any favors. Keep this junk out of the house, office, car, or wherever you spend your time. This will help you avoid triggers and temptations, and you will find it easier to keep your eye on the prize.

Along these lines, plan out your meals and snacks as best you can. By preparing your own food, you will be able to be in control of what you eat when. Try not to eat out or get take out. Restaurants tend to prepare big dishes and large sides, which can mean more calories and fat. As delicious as their meals may be, remembering how you have to squeeze into that outfit may make your home cooking seem a bit more appetizing!

All the while, you have to keep your body moving and try to enjoy your workout as much as possible. If you tend to get bored, or if your body needs a new challenge (which, let's be honest, whose doesn't?), switch things up. Instead of jogging on a treadmill, try out the elliptical, or instead of a hardcore spin class, try lifting some light weights. Don't let your body get used to the same workouts. To see results, change things up.

Don't just put this into action at the gym. Even if you work out most days of the week, sedentary activity the rest of the day can still slow down your metabolism. If you work in an office, walk to your colleague, don't just email them. When driving, always park at the spot furthest from your destination. Aim for a minimum of ten thousand steps per day in addition to your exercise routine. These little things will all add up and make for some extra room in your clothes.

While you're making all of these small changes, there's one thing you don't have to give up: giving yourself a small treat. Even if you're trying to lose a few pounds, you can still enjoy a few bites of something you love. You don't want any of this to feel like punishment. Just keep it to about 150 calories, which can still be satisfying. At the end of the week, the best treat of all will be when you fit into your clothes and realize you did it by moving a little more and eating a little less.

57. How come, when I work out, I get ravenous and feel like I just put back on all the calories I burned off?

It stinks to have an awesome workout and then ruin it by pigging out as soon as it's over. Food is always tempting but never more so than as soon as you've finished exercising. Too often, we believe that sweating our asses off gives us the right to eat more. But, it doesn't!

The reward isn't in racing to the refrigerator. That's why it's important to retrain your mind.

First, try guzzling some water. It's normal that your body is thirsty after an awesome workout. So try to drink a lot of water before you look toward food. Wait about fifteen minutes after you rehydrate and see if the craving for food subsides. If it does, then you know you were dehydrated and, next time you work out, make sure to drink periodically to help ward off the hunger feelings after exercise.

Next, plan smart. Try to schedule your workout so by the time you're done and the hunger sets in, it's mealtime. This way, you're not adding extra calories. It's merely time to eat, so a well-balanced and normal-sized portioned meal or snack should suffice. If you're eating healthy foods spaced every few hours throughout the day, you'll be less likely to be ravenous. That's why it's so important to always stay nourished. It could have nothing to do with whether you worked out; you might just be hungry. For example, if you didn't have enough breakfast, or you skipped lunch, you're going to be starving no matter what.

Then, get in shape! Many people believe that the more out of shape you are, the more likely you are to be hungry after exercise. The general theory is that the body isn't used to burning so many calories. It's been so long since you've been off the couch, it doesn't quite know what to do. Your body goes into a self-preservation mode of sorts and wants to immediately replace the calories it just burned and it starts to prepare for whatever is to come. As you get in better shape, these feelings (like your weight) should decrease.

Lastly, think matter over mind. Sometimes the feeling for hunger can just be your brain playing tricks on you. Many of us associate reaching the end of a workout with a reward—especially if the workout kicked our asses. We have convinced ourselves that if we just burned off a ton of calories, we're entitled to eat some of it back. However, no matter how intense a workout is (unless, of course, you're doing ironmans, marathons, etc.), you don't need to take in more calories, especially if they're unhealthy or empty calories.

There are those times when, no matter what you do, the body needs nourishment after a workout and it's hard to ignore a growling stomach. In these cases, grab a piece of fruit for its complex carbs and fiber. This will help you regain some of your energy and curb your appetite until the next meal. Lean protein is also great post-workout, as it helps your muscles recover. Don't emulate all of the big bodybuilders in the gym, though. Make your protein proportionate to your muscles. Since yours are a lot smaller than theirs, your protein intake should be too. Leave the chicken + protein shake + eggs for them.

Lastly, if you're on a treadmill or an elliptical that has a television, turn off the food channels and cooking shows. While all those dishes are delicious, you made it to the gym for a reason.

Look instead at the incredibly toned people in the gym and use that as motivation.

58. It's hard enough to know what time zone I'm in when I travel. Is there anything that can help with jetlag?

Packing, getting to the airport on time, and through TSA seems like the hardest part of travel. However, the most stressful time on your body actually happens when you're in flight. Once on board, as you fly across time zones, it becomes hard for your body to keep its natural rhythm. Sort of like Elaine's dance moves on Seinfeld—it hears the music and finds the beat, but just can't keep up with it.

Whether you're traveling from NY to LA, Chicago to London, or Atlanta to Hong Kong, jet lag usually checks itself in at some point. It can make you feel sluggish, fatigued, and out of sorts. It does not matter if you're out of town for business or personal reasons; this is the worst way to feel on the trip.

Melatonin is a great aid in helping with jet lag since it works with your body to promote relaxation and regulate sleep. Melatonin can be found in foods including oatmeal, banana, pineapples, oranges, tomatoes, barley, tart cherries, and nuts. It can also be taken as a supplement. It's a great idea to start increasing your intake of this a few days before you leave, especially in the evenings.

Pycgonenol can also be beneficial. This nutrient comes from the bark of pine trees and has been shown not only to be extremely helpful with fighting jet lag, but it can also help support your immune system. In supplement form, studies have shown that 50 milligrams of Pycnogenol when taken two days before and five days after your trip can help avoid these travel-related issues. Although not as easily found in food, small amounts exist in grapes, blueberries, cherries, and plums.

While you're sleeping, resting, or just fidgeting in your seat (as it was made to fit a pre-teen), it's pretty common for those around you to be coughing and sneezing. Vitamins B, C, and E can be great travel companions to help you build up your resistance while you fight the germs flying with you. These vitamins can also help ensure that you don't bring these uninvited companions with you to your final destination. Additionally, when you're flying high, cabin pressure and sitting still for a prolonged period of time can cause problems with circulation, and these nutrients can lend some assistance. Start to add foods high in these nutrients, or a supplement, before you travel so you can make sure your body is properly fueled to handle these situations. They're also important in-flight so put some foods that have these vitamins, like dark chocolate, blueberries, grapes, oranges, and pumpkin seeds in your carry-on bag.

You also have to make sure to drink a ton of water; it's very easy to get dehydrated on a plane. Yes, the bathrooms can make you claustrophobic, and getting out of your window seat is a total pain, but those are not reasons to avoid drinking a lot of water. Besides, getting up out of your seat to pee is a great way to stretch your legs and get the blood flowing again! Avoid sugary treats, sodas, high-sodium snacks, fatty foods, and caffeine, as these can accelerate dehydration. Don't booze it up either. Ideally, you should avoid alcohol when you're flying because it can be extremely dehydrating. If you think a drink will help you relax, then have just one. Besides, you don't want to be that person who has flown all that way just to end up in your hotel room totally hungover.

Once you touch down, it's really important to adapt to the new time zone. Eat at regular mealtimes, even if you're not hungry. This will help to get your body's clock adjusted. Also, do your best to sleep when you should be sleeping and stay awake when you should be functioning. Being a jet setter can be a lot of fun, but if you don't take care of yourself before, during, and after your flight, you might feel like you're standing by the whole time you're away.

9. **When I return from vacation, I feel like I'm wearing a heavy tag around my neck instead of on my suitcase. How can I stop overindulging while still having a great time?**

Vacations are the best. Whether it's adventure-based, relaxing poolside, on a cruise, or visiting family and friends, it's often well-deserved time off. During this break from real life, it's easy to let your healthy habits fall by the wayside. And that's okay. There is no need to turn it into a guilt trip. To ensure you're spending your time making memories and not in the gift shop buying a new wardrobe, there are some things you can do to make sure your clothes still fit when you get home.

Whether you're printing out your boarding pass or packing up the car, make sure to prepare some snacks and/or meals to bring with you. Most sandwiches are a great choice since they're easy to store, easy to eat, and won't make a mess or offend your travel partners with a terrible smell (which is why you should probably avoid a tuna sandwich). You can also bring some baggies filled with healthy options to nosh on. In spite of all your planning, if you run out of the house without them, try to pick up similar snacks on your way. Save splurges for your final destination, though. Skip the airplane food or the fast-food joints you will pass on your drive. You're not going to miss them. You will enjoy the snacks you prepared a lot more knowing you're saving a ton of calories and you don't have to start the trip off on the wrong foot.

Once you get to wherever you're going, choose wisely. Carefully pick your moments to splurge and don't indulge all day long. If you're looking forward to an amazing breakfast or an incredible dinner, enjoy it but make the rest of the day as healthy as possible.

The most common trap while you're away or on vacation is the buffet. By the name alone, they're daring you to eat all that you can. Make it a double dare and don't. Take a lap around and survey the options to come up with a strategy. Once you know what you want, put it all on a smaller plate. That will help you limit your portion size and make sure your eyes aren't bigger than your stomach. If you finish what is on your plate and you're still hungry, it's okay to go up again because you didn't go crazy the first time. You might even find you're too lazy to return to the buffet, so feeling like a beach bum may work in your favor.

During a breakfast buffet, have a piece of fruit instead of fruit juice. Stick to a slice of french toast, a waffle, or a pancake (you don't need a stack). There's no reason to carb-o-load. Make sure to include eggs, yogurts, and other proteins too. Similarly, for a dinner buffet, choose mostly lean proteins and vegetables. Leave the stale rolls for someone else and try to make the pasta, potato, or rice your side and not the main event. You'll be getting the most for your money since the meats are the most costly dishes anyway.

Alcohol is the other obstacle when you're out of town. Getting the time off and leaving some of your responsibilities at home is reason enough to make a few toasts, so chances are you're going to be drinking more than usual. If this sounds like you, try to limit the amount of drinks with syrups, sodas, fruit juices, and mixers. We would never tell you to eliminate all the refreshing tropical drinks if you're somewhere warm, but instead of having multiple cocktails, have one. Then switch to a glass of wine, a mojito, light beer, or use club soda with your spirit of choice.

If your vacation involves staying with a relative, meals can be dicey. You are in their home, so it can get a bit complicated.

If you're not a fan of what they've prepared or if you don't like what they have in the house, offer to go food shopping and stock the house with items you both like. They're being very generous having you as a guest, so this gesture will go a long way for everybody.

No matter where you are, take time to enjoy it. Experiment with the local fare because who knows when you're coming back. Always take advantage of being someplace other than at home and enjoy the great flavors and delicacies of wherever you are. Just pick and choose your spots to indulge. As great as the trip may be, always keep in mind that you don't want your friends and family joking about you having to pay the extra weight fee on the way home.

60. How many hours before bed should I stop eating in order to avoid a nightmare on the scale when I wake up?

It's not about how many hours before bed you stop eating, but rather the total amount of calories consumed over the course of a day. Think of your credit card bill—it's not each receipt that makes you break out in a cold sweat, but rather the sum of all your purchases when you get your monthly statement. In both cases, it's a good idea to set a budget.

The reason most people tend to think they put on weight due to night eating is because of the types of foods they are picking. Rarely are they reaching for a bag of baby carrots or vegetables. Late-night snacking usually involves indulging in all sorts of things—chips, popcorn, chocolate, cookies, or sometimes whatever you can get your hands on (you know what you eat). It's these types of foods that will make you gain weight, regardless of the time of day. People are just normally more prone to eating junk at night.

Why? The answer is often found by taking a look at what you ate during the day. Did you wait too long to eat breakfast? Did you have enough satisfying food? Go too long between meals? Answering yes to any of these questions can cause snacking at night and get you into a bad routine. You're not eating badly because it's nighttime; you're eating badly because your hunger is catching up with you.

If you tend to graze at night, it's also important to determine if you are hungry or just eating out of boredom. If you're only eating because you don't know what else to do, distract yourself. You must have a good book to read, a TV show to watch, or a friend to catch up with. If it is hunger, then eat something real. Stick to lighter options and avoid anything fried, greasy, or full of fat, since these foods are harder to digest and won't sit well in your stomach. As you're about to lie down for (hopefully) eight hours, you'll also want to stay away from spicy foods, as they can also irritate your stomach.

Two caveats: first, don't give yourself a cut-off time to stop eating. When people put a set time on themselves, like "I have to stop eating by 7 or 8 p.m.," it can actually trigger them to overeat or indulge. We all want what we can't have and, when we are too strict with ourselves, it can backfire. Just make a general rule throughout the day to eat only when you're hungry and, no matter the time, make smart choices.

Second, if you have reflux, you should stop eating about three hours before bed. You'll want to stay upright for a while so you can digest your dinner properly and not end up with a bad stomach or burping up what you just ate.

Eating before bed isn't the problem; it's what you do from the time you wake up until the time you go to bed that matters the most. Say good-night to bad eating habits and you might just find your body will start looking like the stuff dreams are made of.

61. Feeling bloated is the worst. Are there foods that can prevent this so people stop thinking I'm pregnant?

You know you're bloated when your belly turns to jelly and your ankles turn to cankles. It's as if all the fluid in your body is on display for the world to see. So, how do you get rid of the dreaded bloat?

First thing to do is drink plenty of water. Contrary to what you may think, water didn't get you into this mess, but it can help you get out of it. The more dehydrated you are, the more likely your body will be to retain water. As you begin to rehydrate, your body will flush everything out and your stomach should go back to its regular size. In addition to just drinking lots of fluids, there are plenty of fruits and vegetables packed with water. Try to include cucumbers, celery, tomatoes, grapefruit, and watermelon in your diet. They can be helpful in taking away some of the puff.

In addition to increasing your water intake, you should also look for foods that are low in sodium. By decreasing your sodium intake, your body will retain less water. Also pick foods high in potassium (like bananas, beans, leafy greens, and potatoes) as they can counteract the effects of sodium. You probably learned about the sodium-potassium pump in science class (although who could blame you if you forgot). However, once upon a time, you knew that when potassium comes in to the cell, the sodium says "peace out."

Fiber-rich foods can also help deflate your belly. These can include whole grain breads, oatmeal, brown rice, lentils, beans, artichokes, cherries, berries, pears, and apples. However, when increasing fiber in your diet, make sure to do so in a slow and steady fashion so that your body gets used to it. You'll also need to drink plenty of water so the fiber can absorb it. If you introduce these fiber-rich foods too quickly, and do so without increasing your water intake, you may get gassy, crampy, or even end up constipated. This will only back up things even more, and getting bloated is a sure thing.

Other foods or seasonings to include in your diet are rosemary, turmeric, peppermint, and ginger as these can all help with digestion and bloating. Eating foods with probiotics or taking a probiotic supplement can be extremely helpful, too. These "good" bacteria can help your digestive system and keep the bad bacteria from taking over.

Avoid gassy and fatty foods for the obvious reasons. Cut out gum, sodas, sugar-free candies and snacks, and limit your alcohol. Eat slowly and frequently throughout the day and get your body moving so the gas doesn't get too comfortable. Passing gas may be silent and deadly, but it might help you get some relief.

62. **What should I eat before sex to get me in the mood and keep me going?**

The most important thing before sex is to eat enough to sustain you so you can last and enjoy the experience. It's also important to feel hot and sexy because, if you're not feeling your best, chances are the sex won't be the best either. To set the mood, try to eat healthy and make sure to drink lots of water to keep you hydrated (but not too much where you have to pee constantly because that's sure to ruin the mood). Make sure you are satisfied so your stomach doesn't growl but don't eat too big a meal where you feel gross, full, and bloated (not sexy!). Bananas are also great a few hours before sex as they can help with stamina, endurance, and even prevent muscle spasms. (Nothing is worse than a cramp during sex—well, maybe some things are worse but that's another book.)

There are, of course, the foods that have long been known as aphrodisiacs. Chocolate contains chemicals associated with pleasure and being in love, while red wine has properties that help with libido as well as those that can help keep the blood flowing. Oysters are high in zinc, which the body needs to produce testosterone. If you don't love oysters, you can always eat nuts, turkey, brown rice, and beans, which all also have zinc.

Asparagus has been known to be beneficial to both men and women because of the folate, which helps with orgasms, but may not leave you with, how do we put this, a "good taste."

Try to avoid foods that leave you gassy, bloated, and tired or those that give you bad breath or make you smelly. So save beans, broccoli, and onions for a day when your beau is out of town or when you know there will be no nooky. Salty foods should also be kept to a minimum as they can inhibit blood flow, which can make reaching an "O" a no. Finally, while some people feel like they need alcohol to get in the mood or lose their inhibitions, it can actually be a deterrent, leaving you (and potentially some of his important parts) sleepy.

Bottom line (pun intended) is to make sure you are well nourished for a great night of passion. Don't worry about the calories because, if you're doing it right, you should burn them all off!

3. **I'm tired of feeling tired. What can I do to lose the urge to snooze?**

In a world where we're constantly connected, it's hard to turn it off. Add family, friends, work pressures, personal issues, and a fixation with social media to the mix, and it's amazing any of us get any sleep at all! Life absolutely does get in the way of catching some zzzz's.

To counteract this, start incorporating calcium and magnesium, as they can help with sleep. This is the reason many people tell you to have a warm glass of milk before bedtime. It's also why some people choose to take supplements containing these nutrients at the end of their day because they can help them relax as they drift off to sleep.

Also try increasing the amount of iron in your diet with foods such as dark leafy greens, prunes, cereals, skinless chicken, lean red meat, and turkey. You can also try beans and lentils as well as iron-fortified foods. Iron helps carry oxygen from the blood to your body's organs and muscles and is integral to the body functioning properly. When incorporating iron into your diet, make sure you are also increasing your level of vitamin C, since it can help with the absorption of iron. Try pairing oranges, strawberries, broccoli, cantaloupe, tomato, mangos, and/or grapefruits with your iron-rich food.

In addition to eating a diet rich in these nutrients, you can also consider a specialized supplement geared toward promoting restful sleep. Look for nutrients like L-tryptophan, melatonin, hops, and Valerian root.

While we know you've heard it all before, it does bear repeating that you should also make sure to eat small, healthy meals throughout the day. Your blood sugar will remain stable, which will prevent dips and/or crashes. This should help keep your energy up during the day and help you rest at night. Stay well hydrated since not drinking enough can cause you to feel more tired. Before bedtime, you can also try incorporating a cup of decaffeinated hot tea, like chamomile, which has been shown to help with sleep. Avoid caffeinated drinks, alcohol, and foods high in sugar close to bedtime since those can all keep you up.

All of this pillow talk should help ensure that instead of staring at the ceiling, counting sheep, or stalking an ex on Facebook at 3 a.m., you'll be drifting off to a fabulous night's sleep.

4. I swore I would never drink again after my last hangover, but I lied. What should I know that I obviously haven't mastered yet?

The only foolproof way to avoid a hangover is to avoid alcohol. But for most of us, that's unlikely. Even though many of us have sworn off alcohol after some rough nights and even rougher mornings, we usually find ourselves with another drink in hand in the days and weeks that follow. If that sounds like you, try these tips to help prevent a hangover or, at the very least, minimize the effects of one.

- Make sure to drink lots of water before, during, and after boozing. Also, it's a good idea to include drinking beverages high in electrolytes that can help with dehydration and rehydration.
- Never go out with an empty stomach. Eat before you head out for the night and try to make healthy choices. Try to stick to foods full of nutrients since those are better at absorbing the alcohol, which will help lessen the hated hangover.
- Stay away from greasy and heavy foods! Grilled cheese sandwiches, burgers, and fries will not be kind to you. While they can be a splurge-worthy treat once in a while, that shouldn't include having them on a big night out. Not only will they

probably make you feel a bit gross, but the alcohol may not mix well with all that grease in your stomach.

- B and C vitamins get depleted from the body with alcohol, so replenishing those after you drink may help with some common hangover issues. Some suggest you load up on them before you go out, as well as the morning after, but this is a personal preference. Have foods like fruits and veggies, as well as chicken, turkey, seafood, beans, and lentils as part of your pre-party meal. If you take a daily multivitamin, these nutrients are usually included in the formula.

If you hit the night hard and the morning comes with an overwhelming feeling you might have to puke, don't pull the shades down and sleep the day away. Get up, get active, and sweat it out. Go for a walk, hit the gym, or take a spin class (only if you're stable enough so you don't fall off the bike), as that will help you feel better and get rid of some of the toxins from the night before. If only you could forget about drunk dialing just as fast.

65. It's so frustrating! Why do men lose weight faster than women?

Not only do women usually earn three-quarters less than a man, but the same gender inequality extends to the scale. Women try and try to take off weight, but the pounds tend to come off v-e-r-y slowly, from a half pound per week to two pounds per week (if they're lucky). When a man tries to lose weight, it seems that once he makes the decision, it just falls off and boom—the scale moves five to ten pounds in a week. The difference can be so aggravating that it can lead to jealousy, fights, breakups, and even in-house gender wars.

Are men just luckier or is there a reason behind this inequality? Science seems to be the answer, so men shouldn't run out for a Powerball ticket just yet. Men, due to their anatomy and their levels of testosterone, tend to be more muscular. Since muscle burns fat, this works in their favor. Women, on the other hand, aren't as muscular. Not only is it harder for women to put on a lot of muscle, but since their bodies are made to bear children, they have 6 to 11 percent more body fat than men. This extra body fat makes it even harder to lose weight. Women are at a natural disadvantage.

Besides physiological differences, women also tend to be more emotional. While crying through every Hallmark commercial and the movie *The Notebook* (no matter how many times they've seen it) doesn't seem to be a hindrance, it's when women's emotions get the best of them and they turn to food that it becomes problematic. Whether its anxiety, sadness, anger, or even happiness, women are more prone to eat their way through their feelings. It's not baby carrots they are turning to for a fix. The sugary, starchy, and high-fat foods are most appealing. Sometimes there is just no stopping it.

These points would all lead you to surmise that the second X chromosome is to blame for the disparity between female and male weight loss. However, all is not lost. While men do lose weight faster than women in the short term, long-term studies have shown that it usually evens out over time. If both genders stick to a weight loss plan of diet and exercise, after six months the amount of weight and fat loss is pretty similar. Women just get frustrated that the men in their lives lose weight quicker than they do and, as a result, sometimes give up.

Stick it out ladies! There is real strength in girl power. So, use this friendly competition to make you want it more and don't feel defeated so early on. While it's not a race, it may feel like one. Just remember, losing weight isn't a sprint. You may start out a few paces behind, but just like the tortoise and the hare, slow and steady always wins the race.

66. I get the worst PMS. Is there anything I can do to make it go away?

If you keep saying WTF and OMG and feel SOL when you suffer from PMS, you're not alone.

Other than staying in bed with a heating pad, zit medicine, a box of tissues, and all the ice cream in the world, there probably isn't much to prevent everyone and everything from getting on your nerves when PMS roars. There are things to do that can help temper your symptoms—symptoms that may include being extremely sensitive, emotional, cranky, irritable, and depressed. We know—it sounds like us on a normal day, too!

Although you may feel hungrier than normal, stick to having small meals every three to four hours to keep your blood sugar stable and prevent yourself from overeating. This will help to ensure you keep your hunger in check.

Since you shouldn't be starving, it will be more manageable to give in to some of your cravings without going off the deep end. It's better to eat a little bit of what you want and feel satisfied than to eat a ton of crap you didn't need in the first place. How many times have you ignored your craving for ice cream just to eat a handful of fat-free cookies that leave you unfulfilled and diving for a bag of M&M's? When that doesn't work, you end up with pretzels, chips, and anything you can find in your pantry. At the end of all of this sampling, you're still unsatisfied even though you probably consumed more calories than you would have if you'd just had a few spoonfuls of ice cream to begin with. The key is moderation and being smart.

If ice cream is what you want, stick to a serving size, which tends to be half a cup, and try not to add any toppings. If it's pizza, order whole wheat and only eat one slice. If it's cookies you can't live without, only have a few small ones and avoid eating an entire box or a jumbo-sized cookie. If it's chocolate, go for dark chocolate or chocolate with nuts. Whatever is the key to your current craving, enjoy a little bit of it and don't feel too guilty. The healthy small meals you're eating throughout the day should allow you the luxury to enjoy a few bites of your favorite food.

A diet high in magnesium, B vitamins (especially B6), and calcium is also important; these nutrients have been shown to be of some help with both physical and mental symptoms.

Most of these nutrients can be found in foods including chickpeas, wild salmon, chicken breast, oatmeal, spinach, broccoli, nuts, kale, and lentils.

If you're considering a PMS supplement, look for one that has the aforementioned nutrients in addition to ginger and chasteberry (vitex), as these may help combat monthly issues. Just remember that none of these are magic pills. You need to take these daily (or as directed) and continuously over time to receive any benefits.

If you're looking for a quick fix, there are always the OTC remedies, a good cry, a sweaty workout, or just crawling into bed and calling it a night. Don't forget to tell the world you'll BRB once PMS says TTYL.

67. **Trying to get preggers. What foods can help my egg attract his swimmers?**

While the act of making a baby is fun, unless you're Fertile Myrtle, getting pregnant can be a long and hard road. You'll hear advice from everyone about everything—optimal positions, times of the day, staying out of hot tubs, etc. What most people don't talk about, though, is what to eat. There are some changes you can make to your diet that can actually play a vital role in getting your body into a positive place to get a positive test result.

You shouldn't wait until you conceive to start treating your body like a temple. It's important to make an optimal environment while you're trying so that you can boost your chances.

A general rule should be to eat the way you would teach your child to eat: lots of fruits and veggies, limit the processed foods, stay away from alcohol and sodas, and make sure you're getting enough nutrients.

As soon as you start trying, since you never know when you might get pregnant, stay away from fish high in mercury. This heavy metal can stay in your body for a long period of time, which is not good for you or a baby. Avoid any food that can be tainted, like soft cheeses and processed meats, and stay away from raw foods including fish, shellfish, meat, and eggs. Limit processed foods, artificial sweeteners, and junk food. Try to incorporate some full-fat dairy products in your diet as they have been reported to help with fertility. You should also try to eat lots of leafy greens, lentils, and broccoli as these are all high in folic acid. This nutrient is not only incredibly important to the baby, but it's also essential for the mother.

If you're finding it hard to get all the nutrients you need from your diet alone, especially folic acid, look for a well-rounded prenatal vitamin. This will help fill in any gaps. You're asking a lot of your body to conceive and carry another human for nine months and you have to show it some love. That includes being at a healthy weight. If you're too heavy or too thin, it can affect your chances of getting pregnant. If you smoke, now's the time to quit. You should also limit caffeine and alcohol—keep the party in your bedroom.

While you're knocking boots, there are still a few things that people swear to that have little to no scientific bearing but stranger things have happened. From legs up in the air to a pillow under your hips and from eating pineapple to drinking grapefruit juice, you never know what will help to create your little miracle. As you're focusing on your temperature, times of the month, and even positions, no matter how tedious it all may seem, have fun and remember—you're making love to create love, so enjoy it!

An Extra Scoop!

It's not only the woman who has to watch what she's eating. A well-rounded diet high in vitamins, minerals, protein, and omega-3s are important for both him and her. These nutrients can help during ovulation, circulation, blood flow, fertilization, and implantation. For women, a nutrient-deficient diet can also affect her period, making her irregular and it even harder to get pregnant. For men, lacking nutrients, like zinc and selenium, could lead to unhealthier sperm. So, try making a dinner for two that includes leafy greens, nuts, beans, legumes, seeds, whole grains, lean protein, fish, and fresh produce.

---

68. **I'm pregnant and can't stop eating. How do I make sure the rest of my body doesn't expand like my belly?**

When your favorite carbs, fatty foods, or salty snacks are consumed too frequently and in large quantities, that's when you can start to look eight months pregnant instead of four. While giving into a craving every once in a while is to be expected, especially when you're pregnant, eating for two (or more) isn't a license to eat whatever you want, whenever you want.

Many pregnant women who are of normal weight only need to consume an extra 300 calories per day starting in the second trimester. (Sorry—we wish it was more too!) When you get hungry, remember these extra calories are easy to obtain by adding a healthy snack to your day. In an ideal world, try to have an apple with peanut butter, a small bowl of soup, a yogurt and some nuts, fruit, hummus with pita and veggies, or a bowl of cereal with milk.

In a slightly more real and ravenous pregnancy world, there are also some other creative ways to snack that shouldn't give you a pregnant pause. Go for air-popped popcorn instead of potato chips and get a scoop of ice cream in a wafer cone instead of adding toppings. Rather than eating french toast or pancakes, enjoy two whole wheat waffles. Bake homemade cookies and substitute white flour for whole wheat flour, and use applesauce, yogurt, or pumpkin or prune purées instead of butter and oil.

Even with these substitutions, we know there are times when the nausea finally subsides and your feet temporarily stop swelling that you just want a little treat for carrying this bundle of joy. In these instances, try to think outside of the box and see if you can keep your snack comparable to the "fruit size" of your baby. At twelve weeks, try to have a snack that's no bigger than the size of a plum. At fifteen weeks, no bigger than an orange, and twenty-one weeks no bigger than a pomegranate. During the rest of your pregnancy, keep your snacks between these sizes and don't go overboard. Go for healthy snacks whenever possible and remember, you're more than halfway through your pregnancy, so there's only so much longer to hide in maternity clothes! This should help keep the unnecessary snacks at bay and make sure it's only a bun in the oven and not two loaves on your booty. If all else fails, remember how you got pregnant in the first place, as that's a great way to burn off some of the calories you're adding to your diet.

69. What foods will help me in the loo when I poo?

Constipation is such a crappy feeling and it can leave you in a bind. You want to go, you know you have to go, but you just can't go. Don't get down in the dumps, though. There are some easy changes you can make to your day that should help to get things flowing once again.

Fiber is number one when it comes to going number two. It not only helps in digestion, but it helps to keep things regular too. Adding foods or supplements rich in fiber will help give you some relief, especially since most adults aren't getting anywhere near the recommended daily amount (which, for those between twenty and fifty years of age, is about 25 grams for women and 38 grams for men and less if you're older). Foods high in fiber include berries, whole grains, beans, oat bran, wheat bran, apples, chick peas, lentils, sweet potato, nuts, almonds, sesame seeds, flaxseeds, peas, broccoli, Brussels sprouts, avocado, and artichokes. Prunes also have a lot of fiber and the skin can act as a mild natural laxative, which is a bonus. There are also fiber-fortified foods like cereals, bars, breads, and juices. These can be a good way to get added fiber, but they often contain only one type of fiber. That's why it's important not to count on getting all your fiber from these sources alone. A well-balanced but varied diet, including all of these foods, is your best bet for lightening your load.

If you're not used to eating fiber, you have to add it slowly. Start with a little bit each day. Otherwise, if you use too much too soon, it might cause stomach pains and you won't know if your bowels are coming or going. You also have to increase your water as you increase your intake of fiber throughout the day. The more regularly you hydrate, the better you will feel, because fiber depends on water. Staying hydrated can also help with constipation, so it's a good idea no matter what.

You also have to get moving to get things moving, and squeezing your abs while on the toilet won't cut it. You have to get up and get active well before that. Exercise of any kind can help the food flow through your body properly, and this should help you go with ease.

As uncomfortable as bathroom problems are when you're home, it always seems to get worse while you're out of town. You tend to drink more alcohol and less water, eat more junk and fewer nutritious foods, and sit more and move less. It's also more likely that you'll hold it in and not want to have to go in less than ideal circumstances, stalls with unclean toilets, or an overly crowded bathroom. That's not going to help matters either. So when you're traveling or out of your comfort zone, it's even more important to stay away from fatty foods, red meat, white rice, processed foods, and unripe bananas as they can lead to constipation.

While these tips might help you go more regularly, you'll no longer be spending so much time in the john. You're going to have to find another time to read your magazines and catch up on twitter. All that's left to do is make sure your bathroom is stocked with toilet paper, and do not forget to wash your hands!

The Inside Scoop on Wellness

"You are what you eat. So don't be fast, cheap,
easy, or fake."—Unknown

70. **What are the foods that I think are healthy, but really aren't?**

Things aren't always as they seem. There are plenty of foods that have the reputation for being healthy but aren't. So many of us have been conned into thinking that some of the choices we are making are good ones, but in actuality, they're not.

Dried fruits, apricots, mangos, cranberries, and even raisins are the perfect examples. As the water is removed and the fruit undergoes processing to become dehydrated, it is depleted of many of the nutrients you would find in the actual fruit. Dried fruits tend to be far less filling than a piece of the same fresh fruit, so you're going to need more to get full. They also can be loaded with calories and sugar (which is why they taste so good). One serving of raisins, for example, has approximately 30 grams of sugar—that's more than a Twinkie or even a Krispy Kreme donut!

Vegetable pastas also masquerade as being healthy, but they are pretending to be something they are not. Many times, they're still white noodles with a smattering of veggie powder or purée. Not only are you not getting the majority of the vegetable's nutrients, but you're also not getting the fiber. While it might be true that you can get a serving of veggies this way, it's like saying you're getting a serving of fruit because you ate apple pie. Yes, it might be true but that doesn't mean it's a good thing to do. In both cases, you're also not saving on calories, sugar, or carbs. If you're looking to make your pasta healthier, switch to 100 percent whole grain pasta. Throw in some veggies with a tomato sauce for the nutrients and fiber you were hoping for in the first place.

Veggie chips are just as phony. Marketed as a "better for you" chip, it's still a chip. Just like the veggie pasta, most veggie chips are made from a little bit of veggie powder or purée. They have a similar calorie count as the same handful of regular potato chips and the difference in fat is usually pretty negligible. Don't be naive when you see a product that has the word *vegetable* in front. If you eat them because you like them, that's one thing. Don't get them just because you think they're healthier. They're usually not. Your best bet would be to make them at home. Cut up a few fresh veggies, add a *little* bit of olive oil, salt, rosemary (or your favorite seasoning), and bake them. You will get the benefits of the veggies while still getting the salty, tasty crunch of a chip.

Fruit juices are deceiving as well, since they are often not made entirely from fruit. Most of them also contain a ton of sugar. For example, Motts Original 100% Apple Juice has 28 grams of sugar per serving/8 ounces. To put that in context, Pepsi Cola has 28 grams of sugar per the same sized serving. It's crazy that they are so similar!! Fruit juices also have very little fiber and tend to be packed with calories without much nutritional content.

Trail mix can also be a trap. It's normally full of unhealthy ingredients like sweetened dried fruit, chocolate- or yogurt-covered candies, pretzels, crackers, extra salty nuts, and sesame sticks. Trail mixes can be healthy if you make them yourself using a combination of nuts, seeds and small pieces of dark chocolate. Caution: whether you make it at home or buy it in a store, you must be careful with serving sizes, as too many nuts can add up in calories and fat very quickly.

While vegan products can be delicious and no animals were hurt in the making of them, they are not necessarily low in calories. They can be chock-full of nutrients, *and* they can have a lot of fat, carbs, and sugars. Just like with other products, it's still very important to read labels and not just assume that if it's vegan, it's automatically healthier. The same is true with products labeled *gluten free, sugar free, organic,* and *natural.* A vegan cookie is still a cookie, organic sugar is still sugar, and sugar-free foods can still have a ton of calories.

Low-fat options, like peanut butter, mayo, ice cream, frozen yogurt, and even muffins, aren't always healthy choices as they often substitute chemicals and sweeteners to keep the taste and texture. Sweet potato fries may have a few more nutrients, but they are still prepared the same way as regular french fries. While granola may have a lot of oats, it can also be high in fat and sugar and you have to keep portion sizes in check.

Think of all of these foods just as photos on Facebook from those "friends" showcasing their perfect lives. Nothing is ever as it seems and things aren't as hunky-dory as they want you to believe. Food is no different, as its appearance can be misleading, too.

71. Is intermittent fasting a good way to cut calories? I'm hangry and can't decide if it's really worth it.

Eating is essential to fueling your metabolism. If you want to keep the fire burning, you need to keep putting logs on it— same thing with food for your body. When you completely restrict food to lose weight, it could have the opposite effect, along with other negative side effects.

There are all different types of fasting including the 12-hour overnight fast, the 5:2 diet (restrict 500 to 600 calories for 2 days and eat normally 5 days), 16-hour fast, eat-stop-eat (24-hour fast once or twice per week), the water fast (only drink water for 24 to 72 hours for no more than once or twice per month), and the warrior diet (eating most of their calories during a 4-hour window usually around dinner time). The 12-hour fast is the most reasonable since it's realistic to top eating at 8pm after dinner and resume eating after you wake up at 8am. This shouldn't interrupt the natural rhythm of your body.

While you may see results at first with the other types of fasting diets, you can seriously screw up your body's natural fire to burn calories and you won't get the long-term weight loss you want. As you go through periods of starvation and restrict your intake of food, your body starts to conserve its energy and your metabolism can slow down. It doesn't know when it can next expect nutrients and energy, so it just goes into a state of deprivation. This state lasts until you start adding food back in, at which point your body gets even more confused as it's unsure when the next meal will be.

Your body constantly needs the nutrients from food to function. Without them, problems can arise—you may grow weary, tired, and find it harder to concentrate. Additionally, anytime there's a drastic change in one's diet, hormones can go haywire. This can lead to breakouts, mood swings, and irritability. In some extreme instances, it can even cause women to lose their periods (while we all have our moments where we hate Aunt Flo, getting our periods actually has many benefits like pretty skin, healthier bones, and a younger appearance). It's also just as concerning if you're thinking about ever having a baby. Intermittent fasting can have a negative effect on your body's ability to reproduce, and it might cause you to get screwed (and not in the way that makes a baby!). No amount of weight loss is worth risking that.

To get through fasting, many people turn to caffeinated drinks. These beverages are used as an appetite suppressant to make fasting days easier and to supply some energy. Too much caffeine on an empty stomach can leave you belly up with an upset stomach or even ulcers. It can also be bad for the kidneys and can lead to insomnia (if the fasting hasn't already disrupted your sleep patterns!). You may think you're fooling your body with caffeine, but you're not outsmarting it. Your body knows it's lacking real nutrients and calories.

This is why you will also probably find yourself obsessing over food. How can you not when you're starving yourself for a full day? Most of us already think about what we're having for dinner while we're still eating lunch. These thoughts only get more intense when we're not eating regularly. Fasting could cause you to fixate on food, which may have the opposite effect you intended. You'll be much more likely to be hungry and overeat once you're "allowed" to eat again.

Your gut may tell you that fasting is the best way to lose weight, but that's not actually the case. Your body needs nutrients from food, and there are so many other healthier and less drastic ways to lose weight.

72. Is it worth spending my dough on a gluten-free diet?

A gluten-free diet is *not* the best thing since sliced bread! Gluten is a specific protein found in wheat, rye, and barley. Many people have sensitivities or an intolerance to gluten while others have been diagnosed with celiac disease, which is an autoimmune disease triggered by gluten. Per doctors' orders, these people have no choice but to eliminate gluten from their diets. While some of them have inadvertently lost weight by having to go gluten-free, it usually is because their bodies aren't absorbing the nutrients. Since some people believed that it was the absence of gluten that led to their weight loss, the gluten-free craze began. They were willing to try anything to drop a few pounds. This "diet" quickly became the new version of Atkins. Or is it one in the same? Atkins has people avoiding carbs, and many who say they are gluten free are following those same rules. However, only avoiding carbs doesn't make you gluten free.

Gluten is hidden in many different foods you eat that you may not even be aware of. Just by swearing off breads, pizza, pretzels, and pasta, you haven't completely eliminated gluten from your diet. You would also have to avoid certain dips, canned soups, puddings, soy sauces, salad dressings, tomato sauces, ketchups, mustards, barbecue sauces, and even some marinades.

If you are being careful and have eliminated all gluten from your diet because you've heard the hype and think it could be a good way to drop a few pounds or jumpstart your system, be mindful: it can actually have the adverse effect. It can lead to weight gain and nutritional deficiencies because some gluten-free products are higher in fat and calories than their regular counterparts. They also can contain other additives that are used to make them taste better. By eating only gluten-free foods, you may mismanage your diet, gain weight, and/or screw up your digestive system.

You shouldn't go gluten-free just because it seems like "everyone else is doing it." A gluten-free world is not necessarily a better world. Barring medical issues, you can limit gluten (like you might already do with fats, sugar and carbs), but you don't need to eliminate any subgroup of food to follow a healthy diet. It is hard to remove an entire category of food from your diet without sacrificing some health benefits.

Unless you're very regimented in removing *all* gluten, you're probably not even following the diet properly. You're actually just calling a carb-free diet by another name. While you may think going gluten-free is trendy, it's like putting your bell bottoms back on, and those didn't even look good on anyone in the '70s.**

73. **A *New York Times* crossword puzzle is easier than picking out a vitamin. What clues should I be looking for to solve this dilemma?**

Trying to find the correct vitamin can oftentimes feel like you're playing "Where's Waldo?" With thousands of choices on the market, shopping for supplements can be a mind-numbing experience. Don't panic, though. Finding the right A, B, and C shouldn't take a PhD.

First, make sure to read the supplement facts panel on the back of each box or bottle of vitamins. Does it have the nutrients you want and are they at the levels you are looking for? For example, if you are looking to buy a daily multivitamin, make sure it has both vitamins (like A, B, C, D, and E) and minerals (like calcium and magnesium). Then, compare the Daily Value (DV) levels to other products on the shelf. If most products have 100 percent of a nutrient, and one has 12 percent, you know the latter one is probably lower in nutrients and may not give you what you want. On the other hand, if most products are around 100 percent and one has most nutrients at 2000 percent, it may be unnecessarily high.

** However, if you do suspect an allergy or intolerance to gluten, definitely consult your doctor.

Pay close attention to the other ingredient section; it lists everything else in the product in descending order. If there's anything in there that you want to avoid (like gelatin, food dyes, or aspartame), this would be the place to look. If no or low sugar is important to you, look for that on the label, as well. If you don't see sugar listed, there is none in the product. If a product is sugar free, companies can decide to list this as either 0 grams of sugar or to leave it off the label. While you're looking at the box or bottle, look for any claims that sound outlandish. If something sounds too good to be true, it probably is. Statements saying a product will cure the common cold, prevent heart disease, or cause you to drop twenty pounds in a week are breaking the law, and you should stay away. No supplement should ever claim, or is allowed to claim, that it can cure, treat, or prevent a disease or illness of any kind, so if it sounds too good to be true, it probably is.

It is also important to remember that everybody is different and the right supplement for one person may not be right for another. While some multivitamins may be good for a large group of people, specific and targeted formulas are not always one-size-fits-all. Just like you may wear the same foundation as your best friend, but different colors for your eyes and lips, you may not necessarily need all the same types of vitamins. Variables, such as your age, gender, activity level, and current prescription medications can influence the vitamins best suited for you. Do not be afraid to ask for more information, but don't trust Dr. Google to tell you everything you need to know. If you have questions about what supplements you should be taking, talk to your local pharmacist, a registered dietitian, or consult your physician.

If shopping in a store, ask questions of those working in the pharmacy or vitamin section. No question should be off limits. Believe us; they've heard it all before! Many, especially in health stores or those retailers with pharmacies, have very qualified staff members who are also interested in nutrition. They can be very helpful and can guide you in the right direction. However, don't get persuaded by him or her if they try to talk you into something you don't want. There are usually more than enough alternatives on the market to fit your specific dietary preferences. For example, nowadays there are products you can take in a number of ways: tablets, capsules, liquids, gummies, and powders just to name a few. There are those without sugar, those that are vegetarian, and those that don't have artificial ingredients in them—so if any of this is important to you, don't settle. Remember, if a store doesn't have what you want, there is probably another store nearby that does, or you can always shop online.

The most important thing to keep in mind is that once you buy a vitamin, you have to take it regularly. When you come home from your shopping trip, take the tags off your new jeans, the groceries out of the bag, and put your vitamins in a place where you will remember to take them each day. We promise they won't work if you don't take them!

74. **Why are vitamins so freaking big and so hard to swallow?**

Taking vitamins shouldn't be a hard pill to swallow but they often are due to their size. Many supplements are considered "horse pills" since they are larger than most and hard to get down. Vitamins aren't big just to be a pain in the neck. There are many fillers and binders sometimes added to formulas that help hold the pill together, and these are often responsible for bulking them up. Additionally, certain nutrients actually have a lot of mass so they take up a lot of room, which often leads to a bigger sized pill.

Most mineral supplements are the largest and hardest pills to swallow, with calcium and magnesium being the biggest culprits. To get 100 percent of the recommended daily value, a pill would need to have 1000 milligrams of calcium and 400 milligrams of magnesium. Compare that to 100 percent of vitamin C which is only 60 milligrams and 100 percent of Thiamin (B1), which is only 1.5 milligrams. With these numbers, it's pretty obvious why there's such a size disparity. That's why many multi-formulas will give you 100 percent of the vitamins, but less of the minerals. A pill that had all of these nutrients at their daily value would be at least the size of a golf ball and probably more than one—imagine getting those balls down your throat!

There are other options if you gag at just the thought of taking these huge supplements. If you don't mind most pills, but have problems getting down some sizeable supplements, look for formulas that have smaller capsules or tablets. Know, however, you may have to take more than one each day to get the same amount as one larger pill. Be careful of chopping or cutting them. Some are time-released so altering their form would be problematic and they'll also probably taste terrible. If you have problems with any size pills, take chewables, liquids, and powders instead. With these alternatives, make sure to look at the nutrient levels and compare them to other products on the shelf to make sure you're getting a good amount of each nutrient. Also look at the sugar content and try to pick brands without artificial colors, flavors, dyes, and sweeteners. With these non-pill forms, it's also important to look at the serving size because some require you to take more than just one per day.

Just remember, with supplements, you always want to swallow, not spit. Find a form that works for you so you can make sure it always goes down easily!

75. **Where should I store my vitamins?**

Vitamins want the same conditions as your hair after a blowout—to be left alone, sweat free, and avoid humidity at all costs. Vitamins do their best when it's cool, dark, and dry. They hate heat, moisture, and light.

That's why the most common places people store their vitamins, like the kitchen and the bathroom, are actually the worst places. These rooms tend to get quite hot and humid, both of which can decrease the effectiveness of vitamins. Kitchens also normally have windows with direct sunlight, which can make the room even hotter—not ideal for keeping vitamins in their optimal condition. Refrigerators, unless specifically instructed, aren't always a great place to store open vitamins. While it may be cold and dark, the refrigerator can create moisture.

When you open a new bottle of vitamins, the nutrients in the supplements can get broken down from the elements. So, try to limit the amount of times you open and close it. While this potential degradation won't make them dangerous, it can decrease how long the vitamins will last and their effectiveness. So, make sure to close the lid fully, making sure it's on tightly and completely.

Most supplement companies purposefully use opaque or dark-colored, thick packaging. This helps keep the nutrients protected. Be even more careful where you store your vitamins if you take them out of their bottle and put them in zip-top bags or smaller cases. If convenience is an issue, look for products available in packets. More and more companies are doing this to make their vitamins more portable and convenient. These packets can also help keep them more stable because they stay sealed until they're ready to be used, eliminating any outside interference.

With all that said, try your bedroom or office as an alternative place to store your vitamins. Those are probably the rooms where you need them the most anyway!

76. Why is my pee neon yellow after I take my vitamins?

The most important thing to do next time you go to take a leak is to make sure to take a peek. Hopefully, you have a white or light colored toilet bowl so it's possible to see your pee. Make sure to use the same toilet bowl when you're keeping track so there are no other variables. As you know from different scales, even the slightest difference can change the results. You need to be able to know the baseline color of your urine so you will be able to determine if there is a change at all, how drastic that change is, and note the color difference.

Normal, healthy urine is yellow. The clearer the better, as this is a sign you are probably well hydrated. The darker the yellow, the less hydrated you are and you should probably increase your water intake. However, if the urine is within a few shades of your normal color, it's usually nothing to be too concerned about as there can be some daily variance based on a number of factors.

Once you have established the usual color of your urine, if, after you take a multi, it changes to look like your favorite neon yellow shirt from the '80s, know that you will not self-destruct. Certain vitamins can cause a change in the color of your urine and this is not harmful. Vitamin C tends to change the color of urine to a more orange hue while B vitamins (especially Riboflavin/B2) tend to change the color to a bright or neon yellow. Calcium has also been known to sometimes even turn urine a blueish color—true story! Certain foods can change the color, too: beets can turn your pee pinkish and asparagus can turn your pee greenish (while also probably giving it a distinctive odor!).

These changes are not necessarily a sign that you peed out your vitamins or that nothing was absorbed. If your body needed some B and C vitamins, but not all of them, your body will get rid of whatever it doesn't need. Since these are water-soluble vitamins, the body won't store them, so your systems are functioning as they should be by excreting the excess. It *doesn't* mean you have the world's most expensive urine.

While bathroom humor can be funny, don't ignore changes in your pee if they aren't temporary. If it hurts when you pee, if you are feeling dehydrated or lethargic, or if you notice any other changes or symptoms that occur at the same time, you should speak to your doctor just to make sure there are no other causes.

77. Can foods and vitamins really help enhance my natural beauty?

You'd be hard pressed to find a woman who hasn't tried cucumbers on her eyes, an egg white mask on her face, or mayo in her hair at some point in her life. We all learned early on that beauty doesn't always come from the bottle.

Our external appearances are actually a reflection of what's going on internally. Just like your make-up bag is full of too many products to count, there are an endless number of nutrients that work below the body's surface to help you look as fabulous as you can. If you are lacking these nutrients, your body is going to show it through your skin, hair and nails. So, you may ask, mirror, mirror on the wall, what are the most important nutrients of them all?

Antioxidants are your foundation and can help you regain your natural glow. The most important beauty antioxidants

include beta-carotene, vitamin C, vitamin E, resveratrol, selenium, green tea, CoQ10, and alpha lipoic acid. They are better
than a "gift with purchase" as they are gifts that keep on giving.
They help fight aging, fine lines, sun spots, wrinkles, hair loss
and even brittle nails.

Biotin is also a must-have. Biotin supports healthy skin and
nails which can help you cut back on pricey spa treatments. Its
most important role though is with our hair. Without enough
of it, your hair may start to weaken, break, or even fall out.
That's because, in combination with folic acid and l-cysteine,
biotin is necessary for hair growth.

Collagen shouldn't be overlooked either. As our collagen
production drops after the age of twenty-five, our cells start to
degrade and signs of aging can become more pronounced. By
increasing your intake of this nutrient, you can help to preserve
your youthful appearance.

There are also other nutrients that prove beauty isn't only
skin deep. They work to brighten, strengthen, and add some
vava voom to our looks. These nutrients include omega-3s, calcium, iron, zinc, inositol, PABA, pantothenic acid and amino
acids, like l-arginine and methionine.

If you're looking for foods that can help you get "looks
to kill," there are so many to choose from. Many of these
vitamins, minerals, and nutrients can be found in berries,
grapes, peppers, watermelon, pineapple, green teas, wine,
chicken, nuts, seeds, broccoli, Brussels sprouts, spinach,
tomato, carrots, and beets. To make sure you're getting full

beauty coverage also include seafood, walnuts, flaxseeds, lean protein, avocado, pumpkin seeds, eggs, beef, and whole grains into your meals.

There are also many supplement and beauty products on the market that contain a good combination of these nutrients. No matter which one you buy, look for those that contain a wide range without promising to be the fountain of youth.

You don't have to spend a million dollars to look like a million bucks. These nutrients are priceless and can help you feel and look your best!

78. Are artificial sweeteners bogus?

Although we usually strive for a diet with a variety of colors, this is not the case when it comes to the multicolored packets of artificial sweeteners. While they deliver on the promise to keep the sweetness but lose the calories, these artificial sweeteners can be a natural disaster to your stomach, taste buds, and health.

The most common artificial sweeteners are aspartame (Equal and NutraSweet), sucralose (Splenda) and saccharin (Sweet'N Low). These sweeteners hit a sour note when you learn they may change the way we taste food. The little yellow packet, for example, is approximately 600 times sweeter than regular sugar, the pink packet is about 300–500 times sweeter, and the blue packet is about 200 times sweeter. Who needs that?! With this extreme sweetness, our taste buds have no choice but to react. As they adjust to a new normal, foods we've eaten for years start to taste different as our palate changes. Over time, sweet foods that we love will become less satisfying. It will take more "sweetness" to get our bodies to respond, and we'll need to eat more of these crappy foods to curb the craving.

It doesn't end there. Your taste buds learn to have different expectations of food, and your body yearns for unhealthy, sweet foods. It was probably hard enough to learn to eat your fruits and veggies when you were younger because your taste buds hadn't matured. Now, you're daring yourself to revert to old, bad habits.

Artificial sweeteners themselves don't add any other nutritious value. It's not as if they're high in nutrients, fiber, or antioxidants. They're supposed to be a healthier version of sugar—but they're really just a low-fat, high "other stuff" substitute. It's not just the packets you have to be wary of, you should also look out for these sweeteners in snacks, gums, sodas, diet iced tea, jams, salad dressings, baked goods, yogurt, protein bars, and even some non-pill supplements. "Natural" sweeteners like Truvia, Stevia, and Monk Fruit aren't much better. They tend to be highly processed, are usually combined with other sweeteners (like Erythritol), and can increase your sugar cravings.

Focus your energy instead on cutting back on real sugar instead of eating foods with these replacements. Even though they are fake, these sweeteners can become problematic and even addictive. Just say no to these white, powdery substances.

79. **Are gummy vitamins full of nutrition, or are they just healthier candy?**

Gummy vitamins are very delicious, but lately there have been some rumblings as to whether or not they are nutritious. Available in all shapes, sizes, and formulas, you can walk into any store that sells vitamins and see that pills are no longer the only option. These yummy candy-like supplements are taking over.

The best thing about these gummies is that they've gotten people interested in taking vitamins. It's a fun way to do something healthy for yourself and it seems like a treat. That is also the problem. Some brands rely so much on making sure that they taste like candy that they forget they aren't candy. Not only do many of these vitamins have artificial colors, sweeteners, and dyes, but they end up missing many important vitamins and minerals or do not have enough of these nutrients.

To see if your gummy vitamin has enough nutrients, compare the formula to pills, tablets, powders, or chewables. As the gummy form can have limited space, it's possible that you may only get a few nutrients and at less than optimal doses. So, you may not be getting the nutritional support you were seeking (or your money's worth). Especially since, to sweeten the deal, many gummy vitamins are full of sugar. Some are full of organic sugars, which is still sugar, and still not good for your teeth. Others are full of artificial sweeteners, which aren't necessarily good for your body. All of these sweet ingredients are used since many vitamins and minerals inherently have awful tastes and some formulas take the easy way out. This can result in the formula having a few grams of sugar. Alone, a gram or two of sugar a day isn't going to make a huge difference. But, combine that sugar with the sticky texture and you have a dental nightmare. Together, they get onto and between the teeth and often stay there for a long time. Just ask your dentist or look at your dental bills!

Another thing to watch out for is how many you should take per day. Too often, people assume it's one gummy per day, but there are some brands out there that require children and adults to take as many as six or eight a day! No matter the dosage, don't pop them to cure your craving for something sweet. They are not candy and they shouldn't be taken arbitrarily. You have to be responsible when it comes to how much you are taking or giving to your child, and always follow directions.

With so many options on the market, gummy vitamins do not need to be your candy crush. There are liquids, chewables, powders, effervescents, or even pills if you don't have a problem swallowing them. Your vitamin routine doesn't need to be a trip to candy land—or the only game you'll be playing will be SORRY!

80. I hate feeling broke when I leave the grocery store. Do I really have to buy organic?

We all know there are some items we buy at discount stores and others we'd rather purchase at department stores. The quality and type of clothes and the occasion for which we're shopping usually helps dictate where we buy what. The same can be said of organic, since it really depends on what you're eating or buying.

The most important types of foods to consider when buying organic are definitely fruits and veggies. Pesticides, residues, and chemicals can be plentiful in nonorganic produce, and normal washing doesn't always mean you will rid them of these potential toxins. We look to the Environmental Working Group (EWG) for guidance on this topic, as they have developed "Dirty Dozen" and "Clean 15" lists. They recommend, and we agree, that it is worth the extra dollars if you can afford to buy organic for their "Dirtiest Picks," which include: apples, peaches, celery, potatoes, cherry tomatoes, snap peas, spinach, cucumbers, strawberries, grapes, nectarines, and sweet bell peppers. They also have two honorable mentions, which are hot peppers and kale/collard greens. While organic produce might cost more on an out-of-pocket basis, the potential long-term health benefits should make them seem like a real bargain.

Fruits and vegetables deemed to be cleaner by the EWG and that don't necessitate buying organic are onions, asparagus, cauliflower, cabbage, sweet corn, sweet potatoes, eggplant, avocado, grapefruit, kiwi, mangos, cantaloupe, pineapple, sweet peas, and papaya.

If you don't have access to organic or if it's too cost-prohibitive, try to look for local produce. They tend to be fresher and usually contain fewer pesticides and chemicals since they don't have to travel as far before they end up on store shelves. If neither of these is available, any fruit or vegetable is better than none. Nonorganic fruits and vegetables will always be more nutritious than any processed snack, so stick with fruit instead of a fruit roll-up. Whether you buy organic or not, it's still always important to make sure to wash them completely before eating or cooking. Even if you don't eat the outside of a certain vegetable or fruit, you still have to wash it well. As your knife pierces through the skin, it can come in contact with the pesticides and you can transfer that to the parts you are consuming.

Organic isn't just for fruits and veggies. Organic milk, eggs, beef, and poultry products are recommended since many cattle and chickens are given hormones. If they are too expensive or unavailable in your grocery store, look for hormone-free, cage-free, and/or antibiotic-free varieties. When it comes to seafood, organic is not always the smart choice. Many fish can still contain loads of mercury, PCBs, and/or other pollutants. Try to stick with fish that naturally have less mercury (such as wild salmon and sole) and avoid farm raised. You do not necessarily need to spend the money on organic breads, crackers, and cookies. For these foods, make sure you're buying those made with 100 percent whole grains whenever possible. For more information on whole grains, see page 12.

Don't be suckered into buying anything and everything just because it says organic. It doesn't always mean it's healthier when it comes to snacks and processed foods. While it might mean "cleaner," these foods can still have a ton of sugar, calories, and fat. Pay close attention to the ingredients and the nutrition facts to determine if it's a good choice.

If you're trying to decipher what is or isn't organic, look for the USDA Organic label. These products must have at least 95 percent organic ingredients. If you see a product without the USDA label, but it says made with organic ingredients, know that it is made of 70 percent organic ingredients by weight. Be careful of words like *natural* as that doesn't, by definition, mean organic. It's an unregulated word so don't put too much stock in it.

31. What is non-GMO, and should it matter to me?

The term *GMO* has been cropping up (pun intended!) a lot lately. From news programs to advertisements and food labels, Genetically Modified Organisms are transforming our conversations about food.

While it can get very technical, the basic thing to know is that the foods we are speaking about have been genetically engineered and have changed from their original form in some way that is not natural. You may think, "Isn't it good when things evolve and morph with technology and the times? I can't imagine my life if I had to fax instead of email or had to text on a flip phone instead of doing everything on my smart phone."

Proponents of GMOs agree with that line of thinking. They cite better tasting and longer lasting produce as being possible only due to scientific advancements. Most specifically, they reference the genetically engineered fruits and vegetables that have increased resistance to insects and environmental factors. These advocates also credit GMOs with being able to produce more crops, which can provide more affordable food for the masses.

Sounds good, right? So, what's the problem? Just as many of us use hands-free devices to limit the potential danger we might be getting from possible cell phone radiation, some feel there is reason to be cautious about many GMO foods. They believe there is serious concern about the safety of many of these adulterated crops and that these crops may very well contain toxins, cause allergies, and lead to more severe health problems.

The recent controversy has less to do with outlawing GMOs, as that seems to be a long-term fight; rather, it centers on whether these foods should be labeled. Many feel strongly that they have the right to know if their foods contain GMOs. Similar to the USDA Organic symbol on food, many would like to see a national standard for GMO labeling. Then each individual can decide whether it matters to his or her purchasing decisions.

As of the printing of this book, there are no national regulations, but there are things you can do if you want to avoid GMOs. The most common GMOs are found in corn, soy, canola, cotton, sugar beets, squash, and foods made from or with these ingredients. Since it's not mandatory that these foods are labeled as either containing (or not containing) GMOs, it's not always so easy to figure out what does or does not contain them. Look for USDA Organic labels and those that say

NonGMO Project Verified, as these are the only way as of now to definitively know these products are free and clear.

It is near impossible to completely avoid foods that have GMOs, so don't get too nuts. Without national labeling laws, it's often anyone's guess. It's up to you to decide how you feel about them and if you want to avoid them whenever possible. It's your choice on how, and if, you want to roll the dice. We tend to keep our cards close and play it as safe as we think knowledge is power. However, everyone has to decide what wager they're comfortable making.

2. The taste of sprouted products is growing on me, but are they better for me?

While they initially found their place in health-food stores, sprouted products are now finding a home just about everywhere. Hippies and vegetarians no longer have this secret all to themselves; many people have discovered them and understand their benefits.

A sprouted grain is formed after the grain develops, but before it becomes a fully functioning plant. As a result, these have less starch, wheat, and gluten while providing more vitamins, fiber, antioxidants, iron, zinc, and protein. These grains also have other benefits, including helping with mood, blood sugar, and cholesterol, as well as increasing the absorption of minerals. Many things can be sprouted: from beans to nuts to cereals and bread. These products are filling up shopping carts since many people find them to be more easily digested because the grains are already broken down. This is wonderful for those of us with sensitive and weak stomachs.

While delicious and hearty, sprouted grains can be more expensive, and you can just as easily choose a 100 percent whole wheat grain for many of the same benefits and less cash. If you buy sprouted bread, keep in mind that they don't usually contain preservatives, so you must freeze or refrigerate them. Otherwise, your bread may end up green—and not the good kind of green.

Even though sprouted products can be full of beneficial nutrients, there are a few reasons to be cautious. The different manufacturing processes that sprouted products must undergo can interfere with their supposed benefits. For example, heat and moisture can destroy or interfere with the integrity of certain vitamins, rendering them less effective. Additionally, young children, pregnant women, and the elderly should stay away from raw sprouted products including alfalfa, clover, radish, and mung bean; they have been known to be a breeding ground for bacterial illnesses due to the warm and moist environments in which they grow. So, if you're in one of these categories, make sure all raw sprouted products are cooked thoroughly.

83. I've heard I should always look for fortified and enriched foods. Are they really healthier?

If you like getting more for your money (and who doesn't?), you would think buying fortified and enriched foods would be the best deal around, but beware! You have to make sure that you don't get duped and you're actually getting a better product.

It's similar to when you go to book a hotel and they make you feel special by telling you that your breakfast is included in the price . . . but then you get to the hotel and realize everyone else got this perk, too.

Enriched foods can be sneaky like that. They boast that they are loaded with nutrients; however, the only reason these vitamins and minerals are absent from the food to begin with is because of the way they were made (usually over-processing). While it sounds like you're getting a bonus, you're really just getting what was in it naturally. It's a replacement, nothing additional. Enriched flour is the worst culprit. Not only is it still missing many of the nutrients it originally contained, but it has considerably less protein and fiber.

Fortified foods contain additional nutrients that aren't normally associated with them. Sometimes this can be great, like when milk is fortified with vitamin D so your body can absorb the calcium. If you're missing key nutrients from your diet, fortified foods can be a good way to fill in the gaps. However, it gets a little shady when companies claim to be a source of certain vitamins and minerals and either have way too much or not enough. That's why it's so important to look at the label to find out exactly how much of the nutrient they are adding. Just because a food may have added nutrients doesn't make it healthy and doesn't mean it's there in any optimal dosage. Fortified foods do not necessarily make them better choices, and you should also make sure to consider the fat, calories, sugar, and sodium levels.

We all like getting a deal, whether it's clothes or shoes or even food. It's important, though, to make sure it's a good purchase, or it's not worth any amount of money.

84. As a former sun-worshiper, how else can I get vitamin D?

While getting some sun does have advantages, including supplying vitamin D, the dangers far outweigh those benefits, especially since there are other ways to get tan (like bronzer and self-tanner) and healthier ways to obtain this powerful nutrient.

Vitamin D is so vital because it aids in calcium absorption, which helps with bone health. Without it, no matter how much calcium you consume, it will not be utilized as efficiently in the body. A lack of vitamin D can have a very serious impact on your bones. Additionally, vitamin D is shown to be an important nutrient in many heart, circulatory, immune, and fertility functions in the body. That's why a vitamin D deficiency has so many different symptoms from which no lifeguard will be able to protect you. Studies have shown that people who have low levels can experience muscle weakness, obesity, fatigue, PMS, depression, and autoimmune diseases—to name a few. Some also say low vitamin D levels can accelerate the aging process. And while we love them, we're not ready to be Golden Girls just yet.

Whether or not you spend a lot of time in the sun, you may think you are getting enough vitamin D, but recent research shows that the majority of Americans are vitamin D deficient. The damage this can do to your body will last longer than any tan line.

There is a bright side: vitamin D can be found in fortified milk (including cows', almond, soy, coconut, rice) or by eating yogurt, salmon, eggs (specifically the yolk), fortified cereal, and sardines (if you're feeling adventurous). You can also take vitamin D as a supplement, either by itself or as part of a multivitamin or calcium product. Vitamin D levels in supplements can vary. The recommended daily allowance is 600 IUs. However, there is a movement to increase that amount, which is why many people take up to 1000 IU daily. You should talk to your doctor about the best level for you and make sure your labs are up to date.

5. Can eating spinach really make me stronger?

Eating spinach can make your body stronger in a lot of ways, but probably not the way you think. The creator of *Popeye* actually made one big booboo when touting spinach for making him "strong to the finich." Spinach actually has about 3.5 milligrams of iron, but Segar (the creator of *Popeye*) believed it was 35. He put the decimal point in the wrong place. A simple mistake any of us would have and could have made (although hopefully not on the SATs). The great thing about his mistake though is that it increased spinach sales by 33 percent. (We only wish our accountant practiced such profitable math during tax season.) Even if it may not be the huge source of iron that Popeye claimed, spinach does have a lot of reasons to flex its muscles.

In addition to iron, spinach contains vitamins A, C, E, and K, thiamin, niacin, riboflavin, and folate, along with calcium, magnesium, phosphorous, magnesium, potassium, zinc, nitrate, and lutein. While this in and of itself is a mouthful, just imagine all the benefits spinach has! Separately and together, these nutrients can be very helpful for good eyesight, strong bones and muscles, healthy skin, supporting your body's immunity, and acting as an anti-inflammatory.

You can incorporate spinach into your diet in many ways. It's definitely one of the most versatile vegetables. You can enjoy spinach raw (like in salads), steamed, or sautéed. It can make a great side dish, mixed into lasagnas, or as part of a gorgeous frittata or delicious omelet.

Spinach has come under scrutiny as it has been involved in recalls involving some pretty gross food-borne illnesses. Abandoning this superfood isn't the answer. Just make sure to wash your spinach with cold water, and wash it very well. This will help in avoiding these problems as best as you can.

If you don't like spinach, or if you want to vary what you eat, other leafy greens have many of the same benefits as spinach. Try kale, arugula, Swiss chard, and collard greens. Kermit may think it's not easy being green, but that's because nothing great ever came that easy!

86. Will eating carrots really help me see better, or will I turn orange?

You know how you start to hate a song when it's constantly played on the radio on every single station? Even though it's a great tune, as soon as it starts to get overplayed, you're done with it. Unfortunately, carrots have suffered the same fate. They are so common that they are often overlooked despite their perfect medley of benefits.

If you take a closer look, you will see that carrots are very important for eye health. Since they are a great source of beta carotene, which turns into vitamin A, carrots are really important for good vision. They also help your eyes glisten by supporting the moisture and mucus membranes and they help distinguish between night and day. Carrots literally help you see the light. Vitamin A is also an antioxidant so it has many other benefits: it can help protect your body against sun damage, aging, and free radicals. It's also integral to so many functions including cardiovascular, immunity, and memory. Those people who don't get enough vitamin A can suffer from night blindness, wrinkles, dry and discolored skin, weak nails, brittle hair, and are more likely to get infections. Carrots also contain vitamin C, vitamin K, potassium, and dietary fiber. Together, all of these nutrients provide benefits that are worth more to your body than any size carat on your finger!

It's important to keep carrots (and carats) clean! Make sure to wash whole carrots thoroughly and peel well. They tend to be very dirty, so try to buy organic if you can. If you like baby carrots better, or prefer them because of their convenience, don't be too concerned with the controversy over them being soaked in chlorine. You've probably swallowed way more pool water, and we're guessing it didn't have much of an effect on you. However, if just the thought bothers you, buy whole carrots, wash and peel them, and then cut them into smaller pieces.

While it would take an exorbitant amount of carrots to turn orange, it is harmless, but possible. So is becoming president. For both, you'd have to work really hard to make them happen.

It's time carrots are shown the love and respect they deserve. They are great, easy, and filling, and they also have that awesome crunch. Yes, carrots have sugar. One serving (which is approximately eight baby carrots) has 4 grams of sugar or 0.5 gram each. Big deal. It's not worth worrying about if you're not eating bags at a time. Besides, who do you know that got fat from eating too many carrots? Carrot cake maybe—but not straight carrots.

Carrots are totally underrated considering the amount of daily benefits they can provide. Don't turn a blind eye to them anymore or else you'll be saying, "What's up, doc?"

87. What's the difference between chia seeds, flaxseeds, and hemp seeds?

Cha cha cha chia! Remember that old television commercial that advertised a ceramic head you could buy, spread some seeds on, water daily, and watch it grow "hair"? Well, fast forward to the present and you've got one of the hottest food trends in the country. Not only are they gaining fame for being gluten free, but chia seeds are also very nutritious. They are often dubbed a superfood since they are high in omega-3 fatty acids, fiber, antioxidants, and minerals. Chia seeds can be eaten raw, but more frequently you'll find recipes that call for soaking them in some kind of liquid. This allows the body to better digest them and get the most from their nutrients. It also helps to make you feel full. Chia seeds are great in yogurts, cereals, oatmeal, rice dishes, and even on salads. There are also a gazillion snack and drink options on the market made with chia.

Similarly, flaxseeds are high in fiber and omega-3 fatty acids. They are also a good source of antioxidants, vitamins, and minerals and are gluten free. If you can't go or are feeling stuffed up, flaxseeds can also act as a natural laxative. So sit back, relax, and eat some flax and you shouldn't need ex-lax!

Flaxseeds are great when the ground seeds are added to your smoothies, yogurt, cereal, oatmeal, salad, or soup. You can also use them in cooking meatballs or burgers or add them to your favorite recipes for baking muffins, pancakes, or breads. Flaxseeds are also available in oils and are wonderful when used as a salad dressing or when drizzled on cooked meat or grilled vegetables. Flaxseeds don't do well with light and air, so if you're storing the seeds or buying the oil, refrigerate and make sure it's in an opaque bottle or container.

Hemp seeds are from the same species of plant as marijuana, but they will not have the same "recreational" effects. They will not lead to the munchies either since they are a great source of protein (with almost twice the amount per serving as chia and flaxseeds). Hemp seeds also contain all nine essential amino acids. This typically doesn't occur in plants, with the exception of quinoa. Therefore, for any vegetarian or vegan, hemp seeds can be a wonderful source of non-animal protein. They are versatile and can be mixed into or added on top of many of the same types of foods as flaxseeds and chia seeds. If you use hemp seeds in baking, you don't have to worry about your baked goods becoming edibles. They don't contain THC, the active compound in marijuana, so you won't get "baked" by eating them. You can get "toasted" with them, though—they are just as delicious right out of the oven as they are raw!

Chia, flax, and hemp seeds are small but mighty. These nutritional powerhouses are a great addition to any diet. Just give them a try. We bet they'll grow on you!

88. **Should I be going green with kale?**

Orange is the new black, white is chic after Labor Day, and kale has been a trendy green food for the past few years. Kale has been featured in magazines, on television, and has the prime spot in supermarkets nationwide. Like other trends, the real question is: does kale deserve this recognition, and does it have the staying power? We believe it does.

Kale comes from the brassica family, meaning it's related to cauliflower, broccoli, Brussels sprouts, and cabbage. Like these vegetables, kale is a good source of calcium, potassium, vitamins A, C, and K, fiber, and iron. It is also high in antioxidants.

When shopping for kale, it's important to know that the color can vary, but that's nothing to be alarmed about since there are many different varieties. If you want a grittier taste, look for firm and deep green colored leaves with strong stems. If you want your kale less bitter, look for smaller leaves in various colors like white, green, purple, or even dark blue green. Stay away from a brown color, as that probably means it's not as fresh.

Kale can be eaten raw or cooked, making it a vegetable that can easily be added to your diet. Don't forget to rinse it well before adding it to your favorite salad, soup, pasta, smoothie, juice, or as a side to your entrée. Try to play with it before you use it—unlike some other things, this will help it go from hard to soft. This can also help stimulate the fiber, which allows it to go down easier. To keep it fresh and make it last longer, *don't* rinse what you're not going to use. Keep it cool by storing it in the refrigerator.

The only big problem with kale has to do with the taste. As it tends to be quite bitter, many people slather dressings or other extras on it to make it tolerable. Too many times, we've seen people trying to be healthy by eating kale, but . . . getting it as part of their Caesar salad? Nothing against Mr. Caesar, but no amount of kale is going to make a Caesar salad seeped in dressing a healthy choice. Nor are kale chips necessarily good for you. Many of the brands you would buy in a store are more chip than kale. A lot of seasoning and additives are usually needed to make it something you'd want to nosh on. If you have the same issue in your kitchen and need tons of other stuff to put on your kale, go back to the basics—there is nothing wrong with spinach and other leafy vegetables if you like those better than kale.

With clothes, trends are only good if they look good *on* your body. With foods, remember that trends are only worth incorporating if they feel good *in* your body.

89. **I'm all out of sick days. What can I do to stop from catching another cold?**

If Grandma's chicken soup can't cure a cold, nothing can! A cold can be very stubborn, and you need to attack it from a lot of different angles.

At the first sign of a cold, increase your levels of vitamins, minerals, and antioxidants. These can help boost immunity and help with fighting off infections in the body. The most important vitamins and minerals are B, C, D, E, selenium, and zinc. Foods rich in many of these nutrients include oranges, berries, leafy greens, carrots, broccoli, tomatoes, sweet potatoes, cantaloupe, bell peppers, nuts, seeds, and seafood. If you don't have much of an appetite, though, you may not be getting the nutrients your body needs from your diet to help it while it's under siege. A daily multivitamin, an immunity supplement, or an antioxidant formula can be good options. Adding in herbs, like elderberry, echinacea, turmeric and ginger can also be beneficial.

Teas can also be helpful. Not only are they filled with nutrients, but just like hot soup, the warmth can help break up the phlegm. These liquids will also help you stay hydrated, and drinking plenty of fluids helps your body flush everything out. You can get a double bonus by squeezing lemons and oranges, which are high in vitamin C, into tea or water.

By increasing your levels of these nutrients, no matter the source, you should be better able to support your body's ability to deal with a cold. Some studies have also shown that some of these nutrients might help decrease the length and severity of a cold.

The best battle against feeling under the weather is to avoid turning to foods or supplements rich in vitamins and antioxidants *only* when you're getting sick. Instead, try to incorporate these into your daily diet and routine so your body has the power to fight germs before they become a problem. The key is to get your body to function properly on a day-to-day basis and not just worry about it as you're reaching for a box of Kleenex.

There are also reports that massages and exercise can help ward off a cold, as they have immune-boosting effects. So, while it's not foolproof, you might as well try to hit the gym and book more spa appointments. Worst case, not a bad way to spend a day!

0. **Even if I'm not juicing, can I have green juice as a meal or a snack?**

Juicing seems to be our generation's version of fast food. When you're hungry but just need to grab something and go, green juices can be a healthy and convenient alternative. If you only have a limited amount of time between meetings, carpools, or errands, grabbing a green juice is better than skipping a meal or going through a drive-thru. Adding one of these juices as a snack or part of a meal can also be a great way to get your veggies during the day.

Juices can be a great source of vitamins, minerals, and antioxidants. While green juices may look the healthiest, you should try to include a variety of colors. This is the best way to make sure you are getting a full range of nutrients from all different types of vegetables, not just from kale, spinach, arugula, and collard greens. Additionally, since juices are really just a mish-mosh of flavors, add in veggies you don't normally eat or like. By combining them with ones that you do, juicing can be a great way to get other nutrients that might be ordinarily missing from your diet.

While most fresh juices only use vegetables, some use many more ingredients than just the stuff you might suspect. That's why it's so important to pay close attention to the calorie and sugar counts, especially the store-bought and premade brands, as they will probably surprise you. For example, Naked Juice Green Machine (100% Juice Smoothie) has 270 calories and 53 grams of sugar per serving. Yes, we said *53 grams of sugar*. The front of the label may state there is no sugar added, but who needs to add sugar when you're already maxing out? This juice, like many others, also has 0 grams of dietary fiber. That's because the process of blending your greens into liquid usually rids them of their fiber. Without it, you may not stay full for as long since you are drinking your veggies and not eating them. You will also not get any protein if you consume these drinks as your meals. A small serving size of veggie-only juices with a side of protein (like eggs, Greek yogurt, or even nuts) would be a better option.

While those who juice often dangle the proverbial carrot about how healthy they are, keep in mind they can drain a lot of the greens from your wallet. These drinks can be pricey and may not be cost effective or worth it. Making them at home may not be much cheaper. At least the professional juicers get to buy their product in bulk, as opposed to you having to buy each and every ingredient, worrying about it staying fresh, and wondering if you'll be able to use it all. The pros also have the benefit of using industrial blenders. The heavy-duty home versions that really pulverize the veggies can cost a good chunk from your paycheck. It's more beneficial, and filling, to eat your veggies in a salad, as a side, or even as a snack.

The best way to stay long and lean like a string bean and not wide like a pear is to eat your veggies as often as possible. For those times when you're in a pickle and just need something to grab and go, stick with a juice made from only Mother Nature's finest.

1. What is an antioxidant, and why is it in my food, my face cream, and my vitamins?

Ever wonder why, after you've taken a few bites of an apple and left it out for a bit because you got distracted, it turns brown and discolored? That process is called oxidation. Oxidation doesn't only happen to fruits; it also happens to our bodies. Caused by things we can and cannot control, like pollution, smog, smoke, alcohol, and even stress, the damage can be both internal and external. To offset this damage, your body needs a well-trained army. That's where antioxidants come in and help save the day.

The term *antioxidant* does sound bad, but these nutrients are actually incredibly helpful. They act as your body's soldiers. Antioxidants work to offset the damage that oxidation does to your cells and, in the process, help limit the chaos in your body. The most well-known antioxidants are vitamin C, vitamin E, beta-carotene, selenium, magnesium, CoQ10, and alpha lipoic acid. You'll be happy to know that you are already taking antioxidants since they are available in the foods you eat, including dark, leafy greens, kale, broccoli, cauliflower, Brussels sprouts, oranges, clementines, strawberries, and bell peppers. They are also available in green tea, chocolate, cocoa powder, coffee, ginger root, and vanilla beans.

Foods aren't the only products that contain antioxidants. Many businesses in the vitamin, skin care, cosmetic, and hair care industries play up the inclusion of these substances in their products, as well. Some believe they work from the outside in, some from the inside out, and some believe in both. All focus on the benefits of antioxidants, which include helping to boost immunity, protect the body against free radicals, work against sun damage, and slow down the physical signs of aging, like wrinkles and dark spots.

There's no substitute for being kind to your body and trying to limit what oxidation you can, so adding antioxidants to your daily routine is a no-brainer. Without them, you are leaving things up to chance. Just like wearing a helmet, a seat-belt, or sunscreen, antioxidants are a great safety net.

What are omega-3 fatty acids, and why do I need them?

While we all know there are plenty of fish in the sea, many of them are great sources of omega-3 fatty acids. These nutrients have been making waves in the health community, as they have been reported to help with heart disease, inflammation, choles-terol, and healthy skin as well as mood, depression, ADHD, asthma, and arthritis. There's pretty much nothing they don't cover.

Since the body can't make omega-3 fatty acids, it's import-ant to get them from your diet. Try to eat cold water, fatty fish low in mercury (like Atlantic mackerel and wild salmon), sardines, or anchovies two to three times per week. From all these sources, you'll get a good dose of two key omega-3 fatty acids: EPA and DHA. EPA works more on the immune system and as an anti-inflammatory while DHA has more of an effect on the brain, eyes, and central nervous system, so it's important to look for a combination of the two. Not only will you get omega-3s from fish, but you'll also get protein and essential nutrients. Don't fall hook, line, and sinker and be fooled into buying farmed fish instead of wild fish. While farmed fish may sound safer and cleaner, they tend to be more contaminated and polluted.

If you are a vegan or vegetarian, it is still possible to get omega-3s from plant sources, including flaxseeds, chia seeds, soybeans, walnuts, tofu, Brussels sprouts, cauliflower, canola oil, vegetable oil, and dark leafy greens. These have another essential omega-3 fatty acid called Alpha Lipoic Acid (ALA), which is converted to EPA and DHA, so you'll still be getting a good dose of these nutrients.

If you don't eat enough foods that are high in omega-3s, if you're allergic to shellfish, or if you want to make sure you're casting a wide net, be cautious when turning to foods marketed as being fortified with omega-3. Some of them (like milk, peanut butter, and granola bars) only have a minimal amount, so make sure to look at the label. To consume the desired amount, you may have to eat or drink a lot, therefore taking in a lot of calories. Also, if you are only eating a portion of the product (like only having the egg whites and not the yolk), you may be losing the part that contains these nutrients. You can consider adding a supplement as an additional source.

If you're pregnant, trying to get pregnant, or nursing, omega-3s are very important for both you and the (almost) baby. They can help with the development of the fetus's vision, brain, and nervous system, help with birth weight, preterm labor, and producing breast milk. It's also important for the mom (or mom-to-be) to get them. Pregnant women actually become depleted in omega-3 fatty acids, as the fetuses use these nutrients to help develop their nervous systems. So, that could be one of the reasons for women experiencing "pregnancy brain"!

Is there something fishy about my bottle of omega-3s that makes me burp?

While omega-3 fatty acids have a ton of benefits, taking the pills can be repulsive. This is especially true when you get that fishy taste—there is almost nothing worse.

The potential advantages to taking an omega-3 supplement should outweigh the few uncomfortable, albeit nauseating, seconds that occur after taking the pill. To not get discouraged from taking them because of these negative associations, we have a few things you can do:

- Try odorless omega-3 supplements as well those specially enteric coated. These may be more palatable and limit the off-putting nature of these types of pills. Some brands are even flavored. While they don't taste as good ice cream, the lemon, orange, mint, and even strawberry flavors should help to mask the fishiness.
- Look for those sourced from alternative types of fish and those that use different purification processes and manufacturing techniques. One may agree with you more than another so don't be afraid to try different brands until you find one that works well for you.
- Take omega-3 supplements with food, which may help erase the taste.
- Use gum, breath fresheners, or mouthwash immediately after taking the supplement, as these should be good at disguising the aftertaste. Think of it as a chaser after a shot. Just be sure

to have them right next to you so you can use it as soon as you pop the pill.

- Try a children's supplement. They usually taste better. Just adjust the dose accordingly.
- Call the supplement company and see if they have samples for you to try to see how they agree with you.

If you're taking omega-3 supplements, look for those that have about 500 milligrams combined of EPA + DHA. Try to buy those in a dark bottle and keep them out of the light. Like most fish, omega-3s like it cool and dark. Once you open the bottle, read the directions, because it will probably tell you to refrigerate the bottle. Refrigerating them may also help eliminate those gross burps. This is a case when being a cold fish may work in your favor!

94. **These body aches are a pain in the neck. Are there foods or nutrients that can help?**

It's very possible your diet can have a lot to do with how you feel. If you suffer from headaches, and not because you're sitting next to a loud talker, there are certain foods you should try to avoid. Some triggers include MSG, artificial sweeteners, processed meats, raw onions, aged cheeses, chocolate, sulfites, nitrates, and alcohol. You should also make sure never to skip meals and to get enough sleep. To try to offset headaches, increase your intake of magnesium, B2 (riboflavin), and CoQ10. You can do this easily by eating leafy greens, quinoa, asparagus, nuts, seeds, wild salmon, halibut, bananas, avocados, dark chocolate, milk, beef, chicken, fish, and eggs, or you can look for a supplement. Caffeine can be a catch-22; it can be very helpful in some cases, which is why it's in certain medications, but too much caffeine, or not enough of it, can lead to a headache.

If your issues are from the neck down, everything that's old is new again. Turmeric, an ancient Indian spice, can help with stiffness, pain, and inflammation and has been widely credited with many healing properties. Ginger has also recently been used by many for its wide range of benefits. Not only is ginger a powerful anti-inflammatory, but it can also help with muscle issues, nausea, and the pains that tend to come once a month for women. Omega-3s, tart cherries, and green tea can also help with inflammation.

If your joints are starting to show your age, try glucosamine and/or chondroitin. Many athletes, former athletes, and even weekend warriors find these supplements helpful. Glucosamine and chondroitin are only available in supplements and can be taken alone or together. If you are allergic to shellfish, though, you should be very careful, as most are derived from them. Look for a vegetarian source instead.

Taking stock of all that you eat and keeping a food log can help you figure out what are triggers and, alternatively, what may offer some relief. Avoid those things that make you feel worse and eat more of the ones that make you feel better. We know it sounds like something Captain Obvious would say, but sometimes the most glaring solutions don't immediately come to mind.

95. **Is there a vitamin that can help take the edge off?**

Whether you're caught in terrible traffic, stuck in a middle seat on a plane, found out your ex has moved on, or everyone and everything is getting on your nerves, who could blame you for wishing for a chill pill! From the mundane to the ridiculous, so much of day-to-day life involves stress. While there are no nutrients that can help turn a bad day into a good day or a stressful day into a day off, there are some that can help make it all more manageable.

Think of the B vitamins as your body's internal therapist (who is significantly less expensive than a real therapist). It's obvious that B6 and B12 are B vitamins. What you must also know, though, is that thiamin (B1), riboflavin (B2), niacin (B3), folic acid, biotin, and pantothenic acid are also B vitamins. When you're feeling stressed, the body looks to these nutrients to help it deal with whatever is making you frazzled. Their purpose is to help you respond to internal and external stresses, which are usually related to one another. As your body deals with all kinds of issues—emotional, physical, and environ-mental—it uses B vitamins and depletes them in the process. Therefore, it's really important to make sure you get enough of these each and every day. Dark green vegetables, chicken, fish, turkey, and salmon are all great sources. If you are a vegetarian, or don't get enough of these foods, try a supplement that has all of these different types of B vitamins.

Calcium and magnesium, found most often in dairy, also work together to help with stress. They balance some of your body's systems, including your muscles and nerves. Selenium, found most often in nuts, can also help support your mood and works well with vitamin E to help you get back to baseline. These can also all be found in supplements, but instead of feeling like you have to buy all of these separately, you can look for a comprehensive multi that contains both vitamins and minerals.

CBD supplements have gained in popularity to help with stress and anxiety. Many have had success with CBD products since they can help with serotonin levels. There are gummies, sprays, oils, tinctures, capsules, and creams—to name just a few. Sorry to tell you, but since none of these contain THC, they won't make you high. However, they can help ease some anxiety.

Although it's possible to eat your way through stress, don't do it with brownies, pints of ice cream, or by taking shots of Patrón. Even though your body may be craving sugar, caffeine, and alcohol, these will actually add to your stress instead of eliminating it. While it probably sounds far less appealing, eating well and taking your vitamins are much better stress-busters.

6. What are probiotics, and is there really such a thing as good bacteria?

Probiotics are the good bacteria that live in your digestive system. There are actually thousands and thousands of different strains of these good bacteria that help your body break down food, absorb nutrients, support immunity, and protect itself from toxins. However, every super power needs an arch enemy, and your body is no different. This is why there are thousands and thousands of bad bacteria also living in your digestive system.

Poor diet, medications, antibiotics, and physical, emotional, and environmental stresses can all cause a reduction in good bacteria and an imbalance to occur. When the bad bacteria take over, you can get indigestion, become gassy, and weird noises may come from your stomach. Did you ever try to pretend not to hear your stomach rumbling when you first meet someone? Pray that your stomach issues would pass so you don't have to explode in a random bathroom? Try to suppress a fart when you're getting a massage? These problems stink . . . literally and figuratively! Probiotics have also shown some promise when it comes to your skin, mood, allergies, teeth and even the common cold.

Probiotics can be found in many foods, including some certain soft cheeses (like cheddar, Gouda, Swiss, and Parmesan), sauerkraut, kefir, miso, tempeh, and kimchi. Many fermented products naturally contain probiotics, too. While yogurts can also be a great source, don't assume they all have probiotics. Make sure the label says it contains live and active cultures. The same goes for frozen yogurt. If it doesn't say anything about their cultures, then it probably doesn't have them. Regardless of the type of food, you can always call the manufacturer to find out for sure.

No matter what you eat, it's hard to get enough probiotics from diet alone, especially with modern processed foods. These foods are frequently stripped of naturally occurring probiotics during the processing. Even eating raw vegetables or fermented foods will give you only a few strains of probiotics, and they often do not have them in any great quantity. Additionally, sometimes whatever they do have can get broken down by your stomach acids. This will result in your intestines only getting a fraction of the total number of what you ingested.

The same is true with probiotic supplements. To get the largest amount, look for enteric coated tablets and capsules (it will say so on the label). Enteric coating will help ensure the probiotics are protected from your stomach acids and stay intact until they reach their home, which is your intestinal tract. If you take enteric-coated pills, you don't have to take probiotics with food.

Look for a formula that has many strains, including Lactobacillus Acidophilus, Lactobacillus Rhamnosus, and Bifidobacterium Longum. It is important to find a probiotic supplement with documented strains. This is the most accurate way to certify the true identity of each strain, and it will let you know that what you are taking has been verified by a third party. You can also look for the registration number (i.e. L. Acidophilus R052) on the label.

You should also try to find a product that has prebiotics. Prebiotics and probiotics are like Batman and Robin, Bert and Ernie, and Peanut Butter and Chocolate. Some things are just better together, and these are no different! Prebiotics are food for the probiotics and therefore give them fuel to work harder and more efficiently. Look for a combination of pre- and probiotics of at least five billion CFUs. Read the directions carefully to see if you should keep them in the refrigerator or at room temperature. Don't forget to check the expiration date, too, as you're dealing with live cultures.

Probiotics are fierce and are the key to a tough tummy. Your upset stomach will turn into belly laughing in no time.

97. Are energy drinks a healthy way to get a boost?

"I have so much energy all day, every day," said no one ever. That's why so many people are looking for an extra boost, and they often turn to energy drinks. Just the name promises a jolt. Whether you're looking for them to provide you with more focus during the day or to keep you going on a late night out, these drinks are just as easy to find as a cup of coffee.

Like your favorite cup of java, energy drinks are full of caffeine. However, many other ingredients like B vitamins, taurine, ginseng, theanine, and/or guarana are usually added as well. They also tend to have lots of sugars or artificial sweeteners so the drink tastes as good as the buzz feels.

While the caffeine and the added nutrients are not the major issue, the number of drinks people consume can make them a monster problem. Most people have energy drinks often and have many at a time. This can lead to excessive consumption of caffeine (especially if you're drinking more than just the 8-ounce size). Side effects from this can include insomnia, nausea, an upset stomach, dehydration, and can even cause your heart rate and blood pressure to increase. In extreme doses, or if you have a real sensitivity to caffeine, it can also lead to some scary episodes, like seizures or strokes.

The scary doesn't end there. If you're mixing energy drinks with alcohol, stop! While the combination of caffeine and alcohol may help you feel less drunk, this can be very dangerous. You might feel more sober than you actually are and you may be able to throw down more drinks, but your judgment will definitely be impaired. This can cause you to make really bad decisions and can cause serious health consequences because you don't realize how drunk you really are. For example, you may not know when to stop drinking and you may get behind the wheel of a car, both of which are very unsafe—especially for young adults who are just beginning to test their tolerance.

Exercising while taking energy drinks can also be very risky. Since you're already at the gym to get a good heart-pumping workout, taking one of these drinks can put undue pressure on your heart. You also may be more likely to become dehydrated, which can put further stress on your body.

If you need to perk up, these energy drinks are not the answer. Try a cup of regular coffee or green tea instead. You should also eat well throughout the day, get some physical activity, make a good night's sleep a priority, and consider taking a daily multivitamin. Take the power back and make changes so that you don't need to depend on these drinks. You can rely on yourself to create your own energy and you'll be raring to go.

98. **Why do I need calcium? Isn't it just for very old people?**

Unless you want to be the lady who falls and can't get up, you should be making sure you're getting enough calcium. Calcium is integral in helping support healthy bones, teeth, muscle (including your heart), and nerves. It has also been shown to help prevent osteoporosis in women and some researchers have even begun exploring possible benefits with weight loss and PMS.

Increasing your intake of calcium alone isn't the answer. Calcium needs vitamin D and magnesium to be at its best. They're a fabulous trio—like Charlie's Angels, The Dixie Chicks, and Alvin and the Chipmunks. Without adequate levels of vitamin D and magnesium, your body won't be able to digest and absorb the calcium, thus rendering it far less effective and less useful in the body.

To make sure you're getting enough of all these nutrients, try to incorporate milk, yogurt, and cheese into your diet, as they have plenty of these nutrients, especially calcium. There are also nondairy options that can provide calcium, magnesium, and/or vitamin D, like oranges, beans, tofu, nuts, broccoli, collard greens, spinach, kale, scallops, Brussels sprouts, bananas, avocados, eggs, and even dark chocolate. Figs and sardines are great sources, too.

If you're not getting enough through the foods you eat, try a supplement that has these three nutrients in the formula for added support. Even though the daily recommended value for calcium is 1000 milligrams, look for supplements that have no more than 500 milligrams per pill. This way you can split the total dose; the body can't absorb more than 500 milligrams at once. Additionally, if you're taking a multi and a separate calcium pill, it's best to take those at different times of the day. Don't be afraid to take it at night either. Calcium at night can help promote relaxation and sleep. There's a reason behind the old wives' tale of having a glass of milk before bed.

Don't wait until it's too late. The time to start getting enough calcium is now, as it can be helpful in both the short and long term. Skimping on it can lead to many unnecessary complications later in life. Just like you are (hopefully) saving money now for retirement, it's important to build up a reserve of calcium. Those years won't be golden if you don't take care of yourself and your body now.

9. **Is there a right time of day to take my vitamins?**

It's hard to say there is a wrong time to take vitamins, as the best time is usually whenever you remember.

For fat-soluble vitamins (A, D, E, and K), if the directions are flexible (i.e., take daily), a general rule of thumb is to try to take them with food. This will help you better digest and absorb them. Many people prefer breakfast time because the beginning of the day is when you're least likely to forget. However, if another time of the day is better for you, then that works too!

If you tend to get an upset stomach from supplements, try taking them close to a meal. This will help coat your stomach and it might reduce any uncomfortable feelings. If you are extra sensitive to vitamins, try not to take a supplement high in B vitamins at night. They can provide a little punch, and taking them too close to bedtime may make it harder to doze off.

If you're one of the many millions of people constantly forgetting to take your vitamins, know you're not alone. Some easy fixes include setting a daily reminder on your calendar, putting the bottle of vitamins by your phone or your keys, or leaving it by your to-do list each day (whether at work or at home). You should always try to take them at the same time every day, on both weekdays and weekends, so it becomes part of your routine. Repetition is key, and this will help make it a habit. It will soon become automatic, like washing your face and brushing your teeth, and taking your vitamins will become second nature.

Specific instructions regarding the time of day you should take a supplement or if you should take it with or without food trump everything, even your habits and preferences. These instructions are always important to follow; read the directions and follow them just as they are written.

Before you add vitamins to your routine, make sure to speak with your doctor, especially if you are on any medications or if you have any health problems. Only your physician will be able to address your concerns specifically.

0. Are dietary supplements regulated? Should I be worried about taking them?

Dietary supplements are actually very regulated. However, it's easy to understand why you might have believed otherwise.

The dietary supplements industry, as a whole, is full of law-abiding companies that follow the comprehensive set of regulations governing it. Makers of vitamin, mineral, herbal, and amino acid products must follow these dietary supplement rules and laws that cover a huge range of concerns including quality control, Good Manufacturing Processes (GMPs), product safety, environmental protection, marketing claims, and labeling. The Food & Drug Administration (FDA), Federal Trade Commission (FTC), state consumer protection agencies, and even the Environmental Protection Agency (EPA) share enforcement authority. However, just like family (or your cousin Joey), there are bad apples in the dietary supplement industry, too. All groups of people, whether personal or professional, include those who are flawed. They may try to cheat the system or even break the law. If they didn't, jails wouldn't exist.

Every family has that one relative. You know, the one family member you don't invite over in mixed company. While he or she may be nothing like the rest of your family, you are still family and you're still associated with one another. While people may never hear about your amazing aunts, uncles, and cousins who are upstanding citizens, you can guarantee that everyone will hear about your cousin Joey and the time he "visited" the county jail.

While bad apples are in the minority, they tend to make the most noise. Just like you don't hear about all the good being done by watching the news, you don't hear about the majority of dietary supplements in the market that are safe and manufactured by reputable and compliant companies. The makers of these products believe in the greater good, and many even go beyond what's required by using heightened quality standards to ensure their products are safe, pure, and efficacious.

In addition to quality and safety rules, there are regulations governing the claims companies can make about a dietary supplement. Supplement makers can't claim their products can diagnose, treat, cure, or prevent any disease or symptom. If a company makes outlandish claims or they sound *very* suspicious, steer clear because (1) they're probably selling snake oil; (2) they are most likely lying; and (3) they are, in all likelihood, breaking the law. What companies *can* say is limited to claims about effects on the structure or function of the body, such as "calcium can help build strong bones." They can't say, "Calcium is going to cure your osteoporosis." These laws not only keep the manufacturers in check, but they also help the consumer differentiate the good from the bad. Avoid any product that is making crazy and outlandish claims. Instead, look for those that focus on supporting overall health and wellness.

Responsible companies acknowledge that supplements are part of the means, not the end. Look for products with third-party GMP certification. These companies are certified to meet, and often exceed, manufacturing and quality standards. Also, know who's selling the product. Supplement labels must include a company's basic contact information on their packaging. Avoid products with minimal or shady company information on the label. If a company and its owners are easy to trace, they're not afraid to have you research them before you buy their products or to contact them at any point.

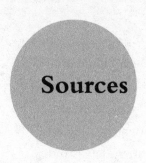

Sources

Introduction:

- IOM, "Health Literacy: A Prescription to End Confusion
  http://www.iom.edu/Reports/2004/Health-Literacy-A-Prescription
  -to-End-Confusion.aspx
- Stahl, P. (2000). Status report on nutrition in the news. *Journal of the American Dietetic Association*, 100(11), 1298-1299. doi: 10.1016/s0002 -8223(00)00362-x

Section 1

1. Should I scoop out my bagel?

- Fox News Magazine, "The Truth About Bagels"
  http://magazine.foxnews.com/food-wellness/truth-about-bagels
- Food Network, "Cream Cheese, Is it Healthy?"
  http://blog.foodnetwork.com/healthyeats/2013/07/19/cream-cheese
  -is-it-healthy/
- SF Gate, "Is Smoked Salmon Healthy?"
  http://healthyeating.sfgate.com/smoked-salmon-healthy-3875.html

3. Should I blot my pizza?

- CNN, "What the Yuck: Does blotting pizza save calories?"
  http://thechart.blogs.cnn.com/2011/04/29/what-the-yuck-does
  -blotting-pizza-save-calories/

4. I'm trying to lose weight. Do I have to give up pasta?

- Medical News Today, "What are the Health Benefits of Quinoa?"
  http://www.medicalnewstoday.com/articles/274745.php
- TODAY, "Guide to Healthy Grains: How to use farro, quinoa and more?"
  http://www.today.com/food/guide-healthy-grains-how-use-farro
  -quinoa-more-1C9002485
- Whole Foods Magazine, "Grain Expectations"
  http://www.wholefoodsmagazine.com/grocery/features/grain
  -expectations

5. Whole wheat, seven grain, rye, oh my! What is the healthiest bread to eat?

- Web MD, "The Best Bread: Tips for Buying Breads"
  http://www.webmd.com/food-recipes/the_best_bread_tips_for
  _buying_breads
- Whole Grains Council, "Identifying Whole Grain Products"
  http://wholegrainscouncil.org/whole-grains-101/identifying-whole
  -grain-products
- Mayo Clinic, "Is multigrain the same thing as whole grain? Which is the healthier choice?"
  http://www.mayoclinic.org/healthy-lifestyle/nutrition-and-healthy
  -eating/expert-answers/multigrain/faq-20057867

6. Are wraps the sandwich solution?

- Eating Well, "Whole-Wheat Bread vs Wraps: Which Is Healthier?"
  http://www.eatingwell.com/videos/v/95385810/whole-wheat-bread
  -vs-wraps-which-is-healthier.htm
- Livestrong.com, "Which Is Better for Your Health: Wheat Wraps or Wheat Bread?"
  http://www.livestrong.com/article/460681-which-is-better-for-your
  -health-wheat-wraps-or-wheat-bread/

7. What's the healthiest breakfast cereal?

- CNN, "How to choose a healthy breakfast cereal" http://www.cnn.com/2012/07/06/health/time-healthy-breakfast -cereal/
- Pop Sugar, "Low-Sugar Morning: Cereals With 5 Grams or Less" http://www.popsugar.com/fitness/Low-Sugar-Cereals-28972028
- 100 Days of Real Food, "MISLEADING PRODUCT ROUNDUP IV: DON'T BE FOOLED" http://www.100daysofrealfood.com/2015/01/ 12/misleading-product-roundup-iv-fooled

8. Lately, it seems there are so many types of milk. What's the difference?

- NY State Dept of Health, "Choose Low-fat or Fat-free Milk" https://www.health.ny.gov/publications/1308.pdf
- Huffington Post, "Everything You Need To Know About Nut, Seed And Grain Milks" http://www.huffingtonpost.com/2014/10/15/alternative-milks_n _5967734.html
- Eat This.com, "Got Milk? Sure But Which is Best?" http://www.eatthis.com/best-worst-milk-alternatives

9. How can I get my cheese fix in a healthy way?

- National Dairy Council, "Cheese" http://www.nationaldairycouncil.org/EducationMaterials/Health ProfessionalsEducationKits/Pages/Cheese.aspx
- Everydayhealth, "Tips for Choosing Healthier Cheeses" http://www.everydayhealth.com/healthy-recipes/cheese.aspx
- Huffington Post, "Yes, You Can Still Eat Cheese And Be Healthy. Here's How" http://www.huffingtonpost.com/2014/06/25/health-benefits-cheese -healthy_n_5523094.html

10. What's all the hype with yogurt? It seems all Greek to me!
- Healthline, "8 Ways Greek Yogurt Benefits Your Health"
  http://www.healthline.com/health/food-nutrition/Greek-yogurt
  -benefits#3

11. Where should I be spreading the love . . . butter or margarine?
- MayoClinic, "Which spread is better for my heart — butter or margarine?"
  http://www.mayoclinic.org/healthy-living/nutrition-and-healthy-eating/
  expert-answers/butter-vs-margarine/faq-20058152
- Cleveland Clinic, "Margarine or Butter: The Heart-Healthiest Spreads."
  http://health.clevelandclinic.org/2014/01/margarine-or-butter-the
  -heart-healthiest-spreads-infographic/
- Health.com, "Butter vs. Margarine, How to Choose"
  http://www.health.com/health/gallery/0,,20509217_16,00.html
- Eureka Alert, "New evidence raises questions about the link between
  fatty acids and heart disease"
  http://www.eurekalert.org/pub_releases/2014-03/uoc-ner031414.php

12. Are egg whites all they're cracked up to be?
- Cholesterol and Health, "The Incredible Edible Egg Yolk"
  http://www.cholesterol-and-health.com/Egg_Yolk.html
- Livestrong, "Does egg yolk give you high cholesterol?"
  http://www.livestrong.com/article/534651-does-egg-yolk-give-you
  -high-cholesterol/
- Harvard, "Eggs and Heart Disease"
  http://www.hsph.harvard.edu/nutritionsource/eggs/
- PubMed. "Egg consumption and risk of heart failure in the Physicians'
  Health Study"
  http://www.ncbi.nlm.nih.gov/pubmed/18195171?dopt=Citation

14. Don't sugarcoat it. Do I really have to give up sweets?
- Women's Health Magazine, "56 Different Names for Sugar"
  http://www.womenshealthmag.com/nutrition/different-names-for-sugar

- Harvard School of Public Health, "Added Sugar in the Diet" http://www.hsph.harvard.edu/nutritionsource/carbohydrates/added -sugar-in-the-diet/
- Jillian Michaels, "Find the Hidden Sources of Sugar" http://www.jillianmichaels.com/fit/lose-weight/hidden-sugar

16. Does being a chocoholic have any benefits, or will it just leave me fat and broken out?

- Cleveland Clinic, "Heart Health Benefits of Chocolate" http://my.clevelandclinic.org/services/heart/prevention/nutrition/food -choices/benefits-of-chocolate
- Women's Health, "9 Health Benefits of Chocolate" http://www .womenshealthmag.com/health/benefits-of-chocolate
- Mayo Clinic, "Can Chocolate be Good For my Health?" http://www.mayoclinic.org/healthy-lifestyle/nutrition-and-healthy-eating/ expert-answers/healthy-chocolate/faq-20058044

18. What's the deal with breakfast for dinner?

- American Osteopathic Association, "The Benefits of Eating Breakfast at Dinner" http://www.osteopathic.org/osteopathic-health/about-your-health/ health-conditions-library/general-health/Pages/benefits-of-breakfast -at-dinner.aspx
- She Knows, "Breakfast for dinner, reversed" http://www.sheknows.com/health-and-wellness/articles/1021237/ dinner-for-breakfast-why-not

19. Can I really eat an endless amount of fruits?

- CNN, "Can eating too much fruit keep me from losing weight?" http:// www.cnn.com/2009/HEALTH/expert.q.a/08/28/fruit.weightloss .jampolis/index.html?iref=24hours

- Shape.com, "Ask the Diet Doctor, Is Fruit Really a Free Diet Food" http://www.shape.com/weight-loss/food-weight-loss/ask-diet-doctor -fruit-really-free-diet-food
- Fruits and Veggies More Matters.com, "Dietary Guidelines for Americans – Key Highlights" http://www.fruitsandveggiesmorematters.org/dietary -guidelines-for-americans

20. Since peanut butter has been outlawed in so many places, what's a good and healthy alternative?

- Greatist, "12 Alternatives to Peanut Butter" http://greatist.com/health/healthy-alternatives-peanut-butter

21. Is Nutella really that bad for me?

- Nutella.com, Ingredients http://www.nutellausa.com/ingredients.htm

22. I'm so confused. Should I be eating sugar-free or fat-free foods?

- Eat This Not That, "Another reason not to eat low-fat foods" http://www.eatthis.com/another-reason-not-eat-low-fat-foods
- Huffington Post, "9 Low-Calorie Mistakes You're Probably Making" http://www.huffingtonpost.com/2013/09/10/common-calorie -mistakes_n_3880665.html

23. Are protein bars a snack food, a meal replacement, or are they just glorified candy bars?

- Eat This, "8 Diet Myths that keep you fat and frustrated" http://www.eatthis.com/8-diet-myths-that-keep-you-fat-frustrated

24. Should I eat before I work out?

- Fitness, "What to Eat Before and After a Workout" http://www.fitnessmagazine.com/recipes/healthy-eating/nutrition/ best-workout-foods/

- Eat This, "7 Foods that will ruin your workout"
  http://www.eatthis.com/7-foods-will-ruin-your-workout
- Men's Health, "Should you hit the gym hungry?"
  http://www.menshealth.com/fitness/eat-before-workout

25. Am I drowning all of my money in those fancy, enhanced waters?

- US News.com, "Which 'Water' Is Healthiest?
  http://health.usnews.com/health-news/blogs/eat-run/2015/04/01/
  which-water-is-healthiest
- Vitmanwater.com
- Smartwater.com

28. What's the smartest way to cook my veggies?

- New York Times, "Ask Well: Does Boiling or Baking Vegetables Destroy
  Their Vitamins?"
  http://well.blogs.nytimes.com/2013/10/18/ask-well-does-boiling-or
  -baking-vegetables-destroy-their-vitamins/
- Time, "The Healthiest Cooking Methods Explained"
  http://healthland.time.com/2013/02/01/the-healthiest-cooking
  -methods-explained/
- Eat This, "8 Cooking Mistakes thet make vegetables less healthy"
  http://www.eatthis.com/8-cooking-mistakes-make-vegetables-less-healthy

29. Fresh. Frozen. Canned. What's the difference when it comes to buying veggies?

- Eatingwell, "Fresh vs. Canned vs. Frozen: Which Is Better?" http://www.
  eatingwell.com/healthy_cooking/healthy_cooking_101_basics_and
  _techniques/fresh_vs_canned_vs_frozen_which_is_better
- ABC news, "5 Reasons to Buy Frozen Fruits and Veggies"
  http://abcnews.go.com/Health/reasons-buy-frozen-fruits-veggies/
  story?id=20683879

30. I want to sizzle in the kitchen. What oil should I use and when?

- Today's Dietitan, "Heart-Healthy Oils: They're Not All Created Equal"
  http://www.todaysdietitian.com/newarchives/021115p24.shtml
- Eatingrules.com, "Cooking Oil Comparison Chart"
  https://eatingrules.com/cooking-oil-comparison-chart/
  https://eatingrules.com/Cooking-Oil-Comparison-Chart_02-22-12.pdf
- Small Bites, "Eight Cooking Oil Facts Everyone Must be Aware Of"
  http://smallbites.andybellatti.com/eight-cooking-oil-facts-everyone
  -must-be-aware-of/
- Lifehacker.com, "Why You Should Have More than One Oil in your
  Kitchen and How to Choose the Best Ones"
  http://lifehacker.com/5992084/why-you-should-have-more-than-one
  -oil-in-your-kitchen-and-how-to-choose-the-best-ones
- PCC Natural Markets, "Choosing the right cooking oil"
  http://www.pccnaturalmarkets.com/guides/tips_cooking_oils.html

31. What's everyone's beef with eating burgers?

- Foodnetwork, "Food Fight: Turkey Burger vs. Beef Burger
  http://blog.foodnetwork.com/healthyeats/2013/06/07/food-fight
  -turkey-burger-vs-beef-burger/?oc=linkback
- Men's Health, "Are Turkey Burgers Really Healthier"
  http://www.menshealth.com/nutrition/are-turkey-burgers-really
  -healthier
- Livestrong.com, "Turkey Burger Nutrition Information"
  http://www.livestrong.com/article/321640-turkey-burger-nutrition
  -information/

32. I used to only eat white meat, but now I really like dark meat. Is it bad that I've ventured over to the dark side?

- New York Times, "REALLY?; White meat is healthier than dark meat."
  http://query.nytimes.com/gst/fullpage.html?res=9505EFDB1E30F
  933A15752C1A9619C8B63

- Fitness, "Food Fight: Dark Meat vs. White Meat Turkey http://www.fitnessmagazine.com/blogs/fitstop/2011/11/15/healthy -eating/dark-meat-vs-white-meat-turkey/
- Eating Well, "Dark meat vs. white meat: which turkey is healthier?" http://www.eatingwell.com/blogs/health_blog/dark_meat_vs_white _meat_which_turkey_is_healthier

33. Is sushi really as healthy as I want to believe it is?

- Fox News, "The Truth About Sushi http://magazine.foxnews.com/food-wellness/truth-about-sushi
- US News, "10 Tips for Ordering Healthy Sushi" http://health.usnews.com/health-news/blogs/eat-run/2013/06/20/ 10-tips-for-ordering-healthy-sushi
- Shape, "The Best and Worst Sushi for Weight Loss" http://www.shape.com/healthy-eating/diet-tips/best-and-worst-sushi -weight-loss

34. Spill the beans. What are some ways to make sure I get enough protein and nutrients if I become a vegetarian?

- Vegetarian Times, "8 Foods Every Vegetarian Should Eat" http://www. vegetariantimes.com/article/8-foods-every-vegetarian-should-eat/
- Greatist.com, "12 Complete Proteins Vegetarians Need to Know About" http://greatist.com/health/complete-vegetarian-proteins?utm_ source=facebook&utm_medium=opengraph&utm_campaign=complete -vegetarian-proteins
- Fitness, "10 Foods Surprisingly High In Protein" http://www.fitnessmagazine.com/recipes/healthy-eating/nutrition/ surprising-high-protein-foods/?socsrc=fitfb15041610

35. I eat well, so what's the point in a multivitamin?

- Energetic Nutrition, "The Importance of Taking a Daily Multi-Vitamin" http://www.energeticnutrition.com/articles/daily-multi-vitamin.html

Section 2:

36. When I go out for dinner, what are the healthiest types of foods at the different types of restaurants?

- Livestrong.com, "Healthy Thai Food Choices at Restaurants"
  http://www.livestrong.com/article/276803-healthy-thai-food-choices
  -at-restaurants/
- WebMD, "Eat Out Eat Smart"
  http://www.webmd.com/food-recipes/eat-out-eat-smart
- Reader's Digest, "5 Healthy Foods to Order at an Italian Restaurant"
  http://www.rd.com/health/healthy-eating/5-healthy-foods-to-order
  -at-an-italian-restaurant/

37. How much weight can I possibly gain following a bender weekend?

- Fitness, "45 Easy Ways to Lose One Pound A Week"
  http://www.fitnessmagazine.com/weight-loss/tips/motivation/45-easy
  -ways-to-lose-one-pound-a-week/

38. All of my friends have been buying cleanses lately. Should I do one, too?

- Shape.com, "4 Reasons to Drink Hot Lemon Water Every Morning"
  http://www.shape.com/healthy-eating/diet-tips/4-reasons-drink-hot
  -lemon-water-every-morning
- Mensfitness, "10 Ways to Detox without dieting"
  http://www.mensfitness.com/nutrition/what-to-eat/10-simple-ways
  -to-detox-without-dieting
- Fitness Magazine, "11 Healthy Ways to Detox"
  http://www.fitnessmagazine.com/weight-loss/plans/detox/healthy
  -detox-diets/

39. What is more important—the amount of calories or the type of calories you consume in a day?

- Huffington Post, "Still Believe 'A Calorie Is a Calorie'?" http://www.huffingtonpost.com/robert-lustig-md/sugar-toxic_b _2759564.html
- Time.com, "You Asked: Are All Calories Created Equal?" http://time.com/2988142/you-asked-are-all-calories-created-equal/
- Dummies.com, "Relating Calories to Nutrients in the Food You Eat" http://www.dummies.com/how-to/content/relating-calories-to -nutrients-in-the-food-you-eat.html

40. Is watching what I eat more important than hitting the gym?

- Huffington Post, "Exercise Vs. Diet: The Truth About Weight Loss" http://www.huffingtonpost.com/2014/04/30/exercise-vs-diet-for -weight-loss_n_5207271.html
- Forbes.com, "The 6 Weight-Loss Tips That Science Actually Knows Work" http://www.forbes.com/sites/alicegwalton/2013/09/04/the-6-weight -loss-tips-that-science-actually-knows-work/

41. Will cutting out dairy help me moo-ve the scale in the right direction?

- Health.com, "Should you be drinking milk?" http://news.health.com/2015/05/15/should-you-be-drinking-milk/
- Dairy Council http://www.nationaldairycouncil.org/Pages/Home.aspx
- Real Simple, "Busting 10 Diet Myths" http://www.realsimple.com/health/nutrition-diet/weight-loss/ busting-10-diet-myths/milk-diets-help-do-they

42. Does it matter if I skip breakfast?

- Mahoney CR, Taylor HA, Kanarek RB, Samuel P. "Effect of breakfast composition on cognitive process in elementary school children." *Physiology & Behavior* 85, 635-645, 2005.

  http://ase.tufts.edu/psychology/spacelab/pubs/MahoneyEtAl.pdf
- SF Gate, "Do You Really Need to Eat Breakfast?"

  http://healthyeating.sfgate.com/really-need-eat-breakfast-2863.html
- Eating Well, "Should I eat breakfast when I am not hungry?"

  http://www.eatingwell.com/nutrition_health/nutrition_news
  _information/should_i_eat_breakfast_when_i_m_not_hungry

43. Will smoothies fast-track weight loss?

- BurgerKing.com, "Burger King® USA Nutritionals."

  https://company.bk.com/pdfs/nutrition.pdf
- DairyQueen.com, "Treats Nutritions & Allergens."

  https://www.dairyqueen.com/en-us/nutrition/treats/
- *Miami Herald*, "Do you love pizza and want to know how many calories are in a slice of pizza? Find out the information about pizza calories here"

  https://www.miamiherald.com/health-wellness/article271357257.html
- DunkinDonuts.com, "Nutrition Guide."

  https://www.dunkindonuts.com/content/dam/dd/pdf/nutrition.pdf

45. Is salt the next four-letter word?

- CDC: Get the Facts: Sodium and the Dietary Guidelines

  http://www.cdc.gov/salt/pdfs/sodium_dietary_guidelines.pdf
- Mayo Clinic: Sodium, How to Tame Your Salt Habit

  http://www.mayoclinic.org/healthy-lifestyle/nutrition-and-healthy
  -eating/in-depth/sodium/art-20045479
- Washington Post, "More scientists doubt salt is as bad for you as the government says"

  http://www.washingtonpost.com/blogs/wonkblog/wp/2015/04/06/
  more-scientists-doubt-salt-is-as-bad-for-you-as-the-government-says/

- American Heart Association: "The Salty Six – surprising foods that add the most sodium to our diets"
  http://sodiumbreakup.heart.org/salty-six-surprising-foods-add-sodium
  -diets/#sthash.y46t0p8b.dpufhttp://sodiumbreakup.heart.org/salty-six
  -surprising-foods-add-sodium-diets/
- Med Page Today, "Study: Salt May Not Be All Bad?"
  http://www.medpagetoday.com/Endocrinology/GeneralEndocrinology
  /49602

46. I'm trying to watch what I'm eating, but it would be a buzzkill if I had to cut out all alcohol. What's my best option?

- Eatingwell, "Taste Test:Light Beer"
  http://www.eatingwell.com/healthy_cooking/wine_beer_spirits
  _guide/taste_test_light_beer?page=3
- CalorieCount.com, Calorie Count in White Wine
  http://caloriecount.about.com/calories-wine-table-white-i14106
- CalorieCount.com, Calorie Count in Red Wine
  http://caloriecount.about.com/calories-wine-table-red-i14096
- CalorieCount.com, Calorie Count in Pina Colada
  http://caloriecount.about.com/calories-pina-colada-i14015
- Calorie Counts, Calorie Count in Tonic Water
  http://caloriecount.about.com/calories-tonic-water-i14155

47. I'm seeing all of these products in the grocery store made from vegetables and fruits. Are they really better for you than the real deal?

- Harvard.edu, "Four Intermittent Fasting Side Effects to Watch Out For."
  https://www.health.harvard.edu/staying-healthy/4-intermittent-fasting
  -side-effects-to-watch-out-for
- Health.com, "4 Reasons Not to Try Intermittent Fasting."
  https://www.health.com/nutrition/4-reasons-not-to-try-intermittent-fasting

48. Why is tea considered healthy?

- Livestrong, "Is Drinking Tea Equivalent to Water" http://www.livestrong.com/article/464140-is-drinking-tea-equivalent -to-water/
- Livestrong.com, "Green Tea Benefits: Cold vs. Hot" http://www.livestrong.com/article/195752-green-tea-benefits-cold-vs-hot/

49. For the sake of those around me, I need coffee! How many cups a day are okay to drink?

- O'Keefe JH, Bhatti SK, Patel HR, DiNicolantonio JJ, Lucan SC, Lavie CJ. "Effects of Habitual Coffee Consumption on Cardiometabolic Disease, Cardiovascular Health, and All-Cause Mortality. *Journal of the American College of Cardiology* 62, 1043-1051, 2013. http://www.sciencedirect.com/science/article/pii/S0735109713026016
- Fast Company, "Exactly how much and how often you should be drinking coffee" http://www.fastcompany.com/3034463/coffee-week/exactly-how -much-and-how-often-you-should-be-drinking-coffee
- Harvard School of Public Health, "Ask the Expert, Coffee and Health" http://www.hsph.harvard.edu/nutritionsource/2015/02/23/ask-the -expert-coffee-and-health-2/
- MayoClinic, "Caffeine: How much is too much?" http://www.mayoclinic.org/healthy-lifestyle/nutrition-and-healthy -eating/in-depth/caffeine/art-20045678

50. Do I really need to drink eight glasses of water every day?

- Cleveland Clinic, "Water: Do you need 8 Glasses a Day?" http://health.clevelandclinic.org/2014/08/should-you-drink-8-glasses -of-water-a-day-infographic/
- WebMD, "What Counts as Water? Stay Hydrated and Healthy" http:// www.webmd.com/parenting/features/healthy-beverages

- EatingWell, "How Much Water to Drink? 8 water Facts and Questions Answered"
  http://www.eatingwell.com/nutrition_health/nutrition_news
  _information/how_much_water_to_drink?page=6
- SF Gate, "Does Drinking a Lot of Green Tea Count as Drinking Water?"
  http://healthyeating.sfgate.com/drinking-lot-green-tea-count
  -drinking-water-10258.html

51. Does writing down everything you eat/drink really help with weight loss?

- Center For Health Research, "CHR Study Finds Food Diaries Doubles Weight Loss"
  http://www.kpchr.org/research/public/News.aspx?NewsID=3

52. In the supermarket, there are so many choices for snacks. What are the best ones when you've got the munchies?

- Consumer Reports, "Are popped snacks healthier?"
  http://www.consumerreports.org/cro/magazine/2013/10/popped
  -snacks-healthy-snacks-consumer-reports/index.htm
- Real Simple, "Low-Calorie Snacks for Every Craving"
  http://www.realsimple.com/health/nutrition-diet/healthy-eating/
  low-calorie-snacks

53. I can't keep up. Am I supposed to be counting grams of carbs or grams of fat?

- Huffington Post, "How 'Healthy Diets' Have Changed Over The Decade"
  http://www.huffingtonpost.com/2015/05/06/2005-2015-healthy
  -diet_n_7209806.html?ncid=fcbklnkushpmg00000032
- Today, "Low-Carb or Low-Fat Diet? New Study Finds Surprising Results"
  http://www.today.com/health/low-carb-diet-or-low-fat-diet-new
  -study-finds-1D80122953
- Shape.com, "Ask the Diet Doctor: Should I Count Calories or Carbs?"
  http://www.shape.com/weight-loss/weight-loss-strategies/ask-diet
  -doctor-should-i-count-calories-or-carbs

55. Are there foods that can help speed up my metabolism?

- ABC News, "8 Ways to Boost Your Metabolism Right Now"
  http://abcnews.go.com/Health/Wellness/ways-boost-metabolism
  -now/story?id=24693412
- FitDay, "Uncovering the truth: Can drinking green tea help with weight loss?"
  http://www.fitday.com/fitness-articles/nutrition/healthy-eating/
  uncovering-the-truth-can-drinking-green-tea-help-with-weight-loss.html
- Health, "The Best Ways to Boost your Metabolism"
  http://www.health.com/health/gallery/0,,20306911,00.html
- Eat This, "8 Best Fat Burning Foods"
  http://www.eatthis.com/8-best-fat-burning-foods

56. What can I do to lose a few pounds so I can fit into my outfit this weekend?

- Popsugar, "Can't get a grip on your diet? Follow these 13 no-cheat recommendations"
  http://www.popsugar.com/fitness/How-Stop-Cheating-Your-Diet
  -36766329?utm_source=health.com&utm_medium=referral&utm
  _campaign=pubexchange_facebook
- Fitness, "45 Easy Ways to Lose One Pound A Week"
  http://www.fitnessmagazine.com/weight-loss/tips/motivation/45-easy
  -ways-to-lose-one-pound-a-week/

57. How come, when I work out, I get ravenous and feel like I just put back on all the calories I burned off?

- Blundell JE, Stubbs RJ, Hughes DA, Whybrow S, King NA. "Cross talk between physical activity and appetite control: does physical activity stimulate appetite?" *Procedures of the Nutrition Society*, 62(3), 651-61, 2003.
  http://www.ncbi.nlm.nih.gov/pubmed/14692601
- Shape, "Ask the Diet Doctor: Busting the exercise-hunger myth"
  http://www.shape.com/healthy-eating/diet-tips/ask-diet-doctor
  -busting-exercise-hunger-myth

- Men's Fitness, "Training Q&A why am I so hungry after my interval workouts?"
  http://www.mensfitness.com/training/cardio/training-qa-why-am-i -so-hungry-after-my-interval-workouts
- Greatist, "Why Your Workout Leaves You So Hungry You Could Eat a Horse"
  http://greatist.com/grow/when-exercise-makes-you-overeat
- Fitness, "Hungry for more: how to manage post-workout cravings"
  http://www.fitnessmagazine.com/weight-loss/eating-help/control -cravings/control-your-post-workout-appetite/

58. It's hard enough to know what time zone I'm in when I travel. Is there anything that can help with jetlag?

- University of Michigan Health, "Jet Lag"
  http://www.uofmhealth.org/health-library/hn-1227005
- Huffington Post, "Got Jet Lag? Food Choices Can Help—And Here's How, According To New Study"
  http://www.huffingtonpost.com/2014/07/11/food-jet-lag-study_n _5564554.html
- Belcaro G, Cesarone MR, Steigerwalt RJ, DiRenzo A, Grossi MG, Ricci A, Stuard S, Ledda A, Dugall M, Cornelli U, Caccio M. "Jet-lag: prevention with Pycnogenol. Preliminary Report: evaluation in healthy individuals and hypertensive patients." *Minerva Cardioangiologica* 56(5 Suppl), 3–9, 2008.
  http://www.ncbi.nlm.nih.gov/pubmed/19597404

59. When I return from vacation, I feel like I'm wearing a heavy tag around my neck instead of my suitcase. How can I stop the overindulging while still having a great time?

- USA Today, "How to eat healthy during your vacation"
  http://traveltips.usatoday.com/eat-healthy-during-vacation-1747.html

60. How many hours before bed should I stop eating in order to avoid a nightmare on the scale when I wake up?
- Jillian Michaels, "Myth, Never Eat Before Bed"
  http://www.jillianmichaels.com/fit/lose-weight/myth-too-late-to
  eat?xid=nl_LosingItWithJillianMichaels_20141215
- Huffington Post, "Foods Before Bed: Foods You Should Never Eat Before
  You Snooze"
  http://www.huffingtonpost.ca/2012/09/07/foods-before-bed-foods
  _n_1861940.html

61. Feeling bloated is the worst. Are there foods that can prevent this so people stop thinking I'm pregnant?
- Well and Good, "9 healthy foods that reduce bloating
  http://wellandgood.com/2013/07/19/9-healthy-foods-that-reduce
  -bloating/#9-healthy-foods-that-reduce-bloating-1
- Fitness, "6 Foods That Fight Off Belly Bloat"
  http://www.fitnessmagazine.com/weight-loss/tips/advice/foods-to
  -stop-bloating/?page=1
- Health, "15 Foods High in Potassium"
  http://www.health.com/health/gallery/0,,20721159,00.html

62. What should I eat before sex to get me in the mood and keep me going?
- AskMen, "Foods to Increase Libido"
  http://www.askmen.com/dating/love_tip_200/230_love_tip.html

63. I'm tired of feeling tired. What can I do to lose the urge to snooze?
- Huffington Post, "Don't Snooze on Nutrition: See How Foods Affect
  Sleep"http://www.huffingtonpost.com/firas-kittaneh/food-sleep_b
  _6762920.html?ncid=fcbklnkushpmg00000030
- Health, "4 Nutrients to help you sleep better"
  http://www.health.com/health/gallery/0,,20707983_3,00.html

64. I swore I would never drink again after my last hangover, but I lied. What should I know that I obviously haven't mastered yet?

- Time, "Top 10 Hangover Cures"
  http://content.time.com/time/specials/packages/article/0,28804,
  2039990_2039991_2040040,00.html

65. It is so frustrating! Why do men lose weight faster than women?

- CNN, "Do Men Lose Weight Faster than Women?"
  http://www.cnn.com/2014/02/20/health/upwave-weight-gender/
- Millward DJ, Truby H, Fox KR, Livingstone MB, Macdonald IA, Tothill P. "Sex differences in the composition of weight gain and loss in overweight and obese adults." *British Journal of Nutrition* 111(5), 933-43, 2014.
  http://www.ncbi.nlm.nih.gov/pubmed/24103395
- PEW Research Center, "On Equal Pay Day, key facts about the gender pay gap" http://www.pewresearch.org/fact-tank/2015/04/14/on-equal
  -pay-day-everything-you-need-to-know-about-the-gender-pay-gap/

66. I get the worst PMS. Is there anything I can do to make it go away?

- WebMD, "Ask the Pharmacist"
  http://women.webmd.com/pms/features/pms-relief?page=2
- Today Health, "Need a Remedy to Help Fight Your PMS?"
  http://today.msnbc.msn.com/id/19405047/ns/today-today_health/t/
  need-remedy-help-fight-your-pms/#.T0VbV4cge8A
- Quaranta S, Buscaglia MA, Meronia MG, Colombo E, Cella S. "Pilot study of the efficacy and safety of a modified-release magnesium 250 mg tablet (Sincromag) for the treatment of premenstrual syndrome." *Clinical Drug Investigation* 27(1), 51-8, 2007.
  http://www.ncbi.nlm.nih.gov/pubmed/17177579

- Livestrong.com, "Can Calcium & Magnesium Help the Symptoms of PMS?" http://www.livestrong.com/article/343742-calcium-magnesium-for-helping-the-symptoms-of-pms/

67. Trying to get preggers. What foods can help my egg attract his swimmers?

- Babycenter.com, "Trying to conceive? Five changes to make to your diet now" http://www.babycenter.com/0_trying-to-conceive-five-changes-to-make-to-your-diet-now_3558.bc
- WebMD, "8 Ways to Boost Your Fertility" http://www.webmd.com/baby/guide/8-ways-to-boost-your-fertility
- Parenting.com, "What to eat to Conceive" http://www.parenting.com/article/what-eat-conceive
- Today's Dietitian, "Improving Male Fertility — Research Suggests a Nutrient-Dense Diet May Play an Integral Role" http://www.todaysdietitian.com/newarchives/060113p40.shtml

68. I'm pregnant and can't stop eating. How do I make sure the rest of my body doesn't expand like my belly?

- Babycenter.com, "What eating for two really means" http://www.babycenter.com/eating-for-two

69. What foods will help me in the loo when I poo?

- WebMD, "Digestive Disorders Health Center" http://www.webmd.com/digestive-disorders/exercise-curing-constipation-via-movement
- Huffington Post, "What To Do When You Can't . . . Quite . . . Go" http://www.huffingtonpost.com/2015/04/07/constipation-relief-strategies_n_7012696.html

Section 3:

70. What are the foods that I think are healthy, but really aren't?

- Shape.com, "50 Seemingly Healthy Foods that are Bad for You"
  http://www.shape.com/healthy-eating/diet-tips/50-seemingly-healthy
  -foods-are-bad-you/slide/40
- Greatist.com, "19 'Healthy' Foods you should reconsider"
  http://greatist.com/health/19-healthy-foods-you-should-reconsider-why
- Eat This, "Diet Experts Won't Eat These Supposedly Healthy Foods"
  http://www.eatthis.com/healthy-foods-diet-experts-wont-eat
- Eat This, "11 Healthy Swaps that Aren't"
  http://www.eatthis.com/11-healthy-swaps-that-arent
- Eating Well, "'Healthy' Kids' Foods That Aren't"
  http://www.eatingwell.com/nutrition_health/nutrition_news
  _information/healthy_kids_foods_that_arent
- Well and Good, "Is granola good for you?"
  http://wellandgood.com/2013/04/30/is-granola-good-for-you/

71. Is intermittent fasting a good way to cut calories? I'm hangry and can't decide if it's really worth it.

- Web MD, "Do Fasting Diets Work?"
  http://www.webmd.com/diet/fasting
- NHS.com, "Fasting: Health Risks"
  http://www.nhs.uk/Livewell/Healthyramadan/Pages/fastinghealthrisks
  .aspx
- Medicine Net, "Fasting Diets"
  http://www.medicinenet.com/fasting_diets/article.htm

72. Is it worth spending my dough on a gluten-free diet?

- Mayo Clinic, "Gluten-Free Diet"
  http://www.mayoclinic.org/healthy-lifestyle/nutrition-and-healthy
  -eating/in-depth/gluten-free-diet/art-20048530

- American Diabetes Association, "What Foods Have Gluten?"
  http://www.diabetes.org/food-and-fitness/food/planning-meals/
  gluten-free-diets/what-foods-have-gluten.html?referrer=https://www
  .google.com/

73. A *New York Times* crossword puzzle is easier than picking out a vitamin. What clues should I be looking for to solve this dilemma?
- NIH, "Dietary Supplement Guidelines, Frequently Asked Questions"
  http://ods.od.nih.gov/Health_Information/ODS_Frequently_Asked
  _Questions.aspx

76. Why is my pee neon yellow after I take my vitamins?
- Cleveland Clinic, "What The Color of Your Urine Says About You" http://
  health.clevelandclinic.org/2013/10/what-the-color-of-your-urine-says
  -about-you-infographic/
- Livestrong, "Can vitamins change the color of your urine?"
  http://www.livestrong.com/article/543711-can-vitamins-change-the
  -color-of-your-urine/#ixzz1mew0HuKp

77. Can foods and vitamins really help enhance my natural beauty?
- Joy Bauer, How Food Affects Hair Health
  http://www.joybauer.com/looking-great/how-food-affects-hair-health.aspx
- Huffington Post, "10 Beauty Foods For Glowing Skin And Shiny Hair"
  http://www.huffingtonpost.com/thrive-market/beauty-foods-for
  -glowing-skin-shiny-hair_b_7192880.html?ncid=fcbklnkushpmg000
  00032
- Eating Well, "5 Beauty Foods For Natural Radiance"
  http://www.eatingwell.com/nutrition_health/nutrition_news
  _information/5_beauty_foods_for_natural_radiance?page=3

78. Are artificial sweeteners bogus?

- Rodale's Organic Life, "7 More Hidden Dangers of Artificial Sweeteners" http://www.rodalesorganiclife.com/food/dangers-artificial-sweeteners
- NY Times, "Artificial Sweeteners: The Challenges of Tricking the Taste Buds" http://well.blogs.nytimes.com/2012/06/11/artificial-sweeteners-the -challenges-of-tricking-the-taste-buds/?_r=1
- Medline Plus, "Sweeteners - sugar substitutes" http://www.nlm.nih.gov/medlineplus/ency/article/007492.htm

80. I hate feeling broke when I leave the grocery store. Do I really have to buy organic?

- USDA, "Organic Argriculture" http://www.usda.gov/wps/portal/usda/usdahome?contentidonly=true &contentid=organic-agriculture.html
- EWG, "Shopper's Guide to Pesticides in Produce" http://www.ewg.org/foodnews/
- New York Times: "Study of Organic Crops Finds Fewer Pesticides and More Antioxidants" http://www.nytimes.com/2014/07/12/science/earth/ study-of-organic-crops-finds-fewer-pesticides-and-more-antioxidants -.html?module=Search&mabReward=relbias%3Ar%2C%7B%221%22% 3A%22RI%3A5%22%7D

81. What is non-GMO, and should it matter to me?

- Whole Foods Magazine, "The GMO Controversy: What You Need to Know" http://www.wholefoodsmagazine.com/columns/consumer -bulletin/gmo-controversy-what-you-need-know
- Non GMO Project, "GMO Facts" http://www.nongmoproject.org/learn-more

82. The taste of sprouted products is growing on me, but are they better for me?

- Whole Grains Council, "Sprouted Whole Grains"

http://wholegrainscouncil.org/whole-grains-101/sprouted-whole
-grains
- US News & World Report, "What are Sprouted Grains?"
  http://health.usnews.com/health-news/blogs/eat-run/2012/11/27/
  what-are-sprouted-grains
- FDA: Growing Sprouts in Retail Food Establishment. http://www.fda.
  gov/Food/GuidanceRegulation/RetailFoodProtection/ucm078758.htm
- FDA: Food Safety for Moms-to-Be: Safe Eats - Fruits, Veggies & Juices
  http://www.fda.gov/Food/ResourcesForYou/HealthEducators/
  ucm082417.htm

83. I've heard I should always look for fortified and enriched foods. Are they really healthier?

- USDA, "What about fortified foods"
  http://www.choosemyplate.gov/pregnancy-breastfeeding/fortified
  -foods.html
- University of Chicago, "What's the difference between 'enriched' and
  'fortified' when it comes to foods?"
  http://www.cureceliacdisease.org/archives/faq/whats-the-difference
  -between-enriched-and-fortified-when-it-comes-to-foods
- Nutrition.About.Com, "What Are Enriched and Fortified Foods?
  http://nutrition.about.com/od/askyournutritionist/f/enriched.htm

84. As a former sun-worshipper, how else can I get Vitamin D?

- Harvard, "Vitamin D and Health"
  http://www.hsph.harvard.edu/nutritionsource/vitamin-d/
- Women's Health, "Why Do you Need more Vitamin D" http://www
  .womenshealthmag.com/nutritionvitamin-d-benefits#ixzz1mf2HpQ00
- Medical News Today, Vitamin D: Health Benefits, Uses and Health Risks
  http://www.medicalnewstoday.com/articles/161618.php

85. Can eating spinach really make me stronger?

- USDA, "National Nutrient Database – Spinach"
  http://ndb.nal.usda.gov/ndb/foods/show/3202
- University of Arkansas Medical Sciences, "Is Spinach a great source of Iron." http://www.uamshealth.com/spinach
- Daily Mail, "Sorry Popeye, spinach DOESN'T make your muscles big: Expert reveals sailor's love of the food was due to a misplaced decimal point http://www.dailymail.co.uk/sciencetech/article-2354580/Popeyes -legendary-love-spinach-actually-misplaced-decimal-point.html

86. Will eating carrots really help me see better, or will I turn orange?

- Reader's Digest, "6 Surprising Health Benefits to Eating Your Carrots"
  http://www.rd.com/slideshows/benefits-of-carrots/#ixzz3czfwY9Z
  hhttp://www.rd.com/slideshows/benefits-of-carrots/#slideshow=slide2
- USDA, "Foods Fact Sheet – Carrots"
  http://www.fns.usda.gov/sites/default/files/HHFS_CARROTS _FRESH_Dec2012.pdf
- UAMS Health: "If you eat too many carrots, will your skin to orange?"
  http://uamshealth.com/healthlibrary2/medicalmyths/medicalmythscarrots/

87. What's the difference between chia seeds, flaxseeds, and hemp seeds?

- Academy of Nutrition and Dietetics, "What Are Chia Seeds?
  http://www.eatright.org/resource/food/vitamins-and-supplements/ nutrient-rich-foods/what-are-chia-seeds
- Tufts, "Should You Jump on the Chia Seed Bandwagon"
  http://www.nutritionletter.tufts.edu/issues/9_3/current-articles/ Should-You-Jump-on-the-Chia-Seeds-Bandwagon_967-1.html
- Today's Dietitian, "What's New in Flax?"
  http://www.todaysdietitian.com/newarchives/050113p34.shtml

- Department of Pharmaceutical Chemistry, "Hempseed as a nutritional resource: An overview." University of Kuopio, Finland http://www .finola.com/Hempseed%20Nutrition.pdf

88. Should I be going green with kale?
- Everything You Ever Needed To Know About Kale http://www.care2.com/greenliving/everything-you-ever-need-to -know-about-kale.html
- Nutrition Data, "Kale." http://nutritiondata.self.com/facts/vegetables-and-vegetable-products/ 2461/2
- BuiltLean, "Kale 101: how to buy, store, & enjoy kale" http://www.builtlean.com/2012/09/18/kale/

89. I'm all out of sick days. What can I do to stop from catching another cold?
- Huffington Post, "The Best Way To Fight A Cold" http://www.huffingtonpost.com/2012/12/11/best-way-to-fight -cold_n_2273083.html
- Mayo Clinic, "Will taking zinc for colds make my colds go away faster?" http://www.mayoclinic.org/diseases-conditions/common-cold/ expert-answers/zinc-for-colds/faq-20057769
- NIH, "The Flu, the Common Cold, and Complementary Health Approaches" https://nccih.nih.gov/health/flu/ataglance.htm

90. Even if I'm not juicing, can I have green juice as a meal or a snack?
- ABC News, "5 Things You Need to Know About Green Juice." http:// abcnews.go.com/Health/Wellness/things-green-juice/story?id= 22849228#1
- Naked Juice, Green Machine

http://nakedjuice.com/our-products/juice/green-machine

91. What is an antioxidant, and why is it in my food, my face cream, and my vitamins?

• Harvard, Antioxidants: Beyond the Hype
  http://www.hsph.harvard.edu/nutritionsource/antioxidants/

• Livestrong, "Benefits of Antioxidants in Skin Care"
  http://www.livestrong.com/article/87141-benefits-antioxidants-skin-care/

• Howstuffworks, "Antioxidants: What You Need to Know"
  http://health.howstuffworks.com/wellness/food-nutrition/facts/
  antioxidant1.htm

92. What are omega-3 fatty acids, and why do I need them?

• Greenberg JA, Bell SJ, Van Ausdal W. "Omega-3 Fatty Acid Supplementation During Pregnancy. *Revue of Obstetric Gynecology* 1(4), 162-169, 2008.
  http://www.ncbi.nlm.nih.gov/pmc/articles/PMC2621042/

• American Pregnancy Association, "Omega-3 Fish Oil and Pregnancy"
  http://americanpregnancy.org/pregnancy-health/omega-3-fish-oil/

• Harvard School of Public Health, "Omega-3 Fatty Acids: An Essential Contribution"
  http://www.hsph.harvard.edu/nutritionsource/omega-3-fats/

93. Is there something fishy about my bottle of omega-3s that makes me burp?

• Livestrong, "Why Does Fish Oil Make you Burp?"
  http://www.livestrong.com/article/471220-why-does-fish-oil-make
  -you-burp/

• Niche Topics, "3 Simple Ways to Stop Fish Oil Burps"
  http://www.nichetopics.info/simple-ways-to-stop-fish-oil-burps.html

94. These body aches are a pain in the neck. Are there foods or nutrients that can help?

- Medical News Today, "Ginger: Health Benefits and Nutritional Information" http://www.medicalnewstoday.com/articles/265990.php
- Arthritis Today, "Olive Oil Reduces Inflammation" http://www.arthritistoday.org/what-you-can-do/eating-well/arthritis -diet/olive-oil-inflammation.php
- Health, "14 Foods that Fight Inflammation" http://www.health.com/health/gallery/0,,20705881,00.html

95. Is there a vitamin that can help take the edge off?

- Greatist, "10 Nutrients Scientifically Proven to Make You Feel Awesome" http://greatist.com/happiness/nutrients-boost-mood?utm_source= facebook&utm_medium=opengraph&utm_campaign=nutrients-boost -mood

96. What are probiotics, and is there really such a thing as good bacteria?

- National Center for Complementary and Integrative Health: Probiotics https://nccih.nih.gov/health/probiotics/introduction.htm
- Huffington Post, "Probiotics May One Day Be Used to Treat Depression" http://www.huffingtonpost.com/2015/04/17/probiotics-depression _n_7064030.html
- Harvard Health, "Health benefits of taking probiotics" http://www.health.harvard.edu/vitamins-and-supplements/ health-benefits-of-taking-probiotics
- Berkley Wellness, "Probiotic Pros and Cons" http://www.berkeleywellness.com/supplements/other-supplements/ article/probiotics-pros-and-cons

97. Are energy drinks a healthy way to get a boost?

- Mayo Clinic, "Can energy drinks really boost a person's energy?" http://www.mayoclinic.org/healthy-lifestyle/nutrition-and-healthy-eating/expert-answers/energy-drinks/faq-20058349
- Huffington Post, "Just how dangerous are energy drinks, anyway?" http://www.huffingtonpost.com/2014/06/23/just-how-dangerous-are-energy-drinks_n_5515647.html
- CNN, "What's in your energy drink?" http://www.cnn.com/2013/02/06/health/time-energy-drink/

100. Are dietary supplements regulated? Should I be worried about taking them?

- NIH, "Dietary Supplement Guidelines, Frequently Asked Questions" http://ods.od.nih.gov/Health_Information/ODS_Frequently_Asked_Questions.aspx

Acknowledgments

Ilyse & Hallie

This book would not have been possible without the enthusiasm of our agent, Linda Konner. Linda, thank you for encouraging us to stay true to our vision and for always having our backs. We are forever grateful. To Nicole Frail, our editor extraordinaire, whose guidance and careful attention to detail helped bring this book to life. We are so appreciative of your patience, especially through our hyphen and spacing obsessions! And to Mike Onorato for his excitement and passion. Mike, we are so lucky to have you part of the *Scoop* team.

A heartfelt thank you to Ronni Rich, Rochelle Polsky, and Toni Wiener for going above and beyond in reading (and rereading) every word in this book. Your edits were always spot on, especially when pointing out our overuse of commas or particular words and phrases. To Mike, Evan, Barrie, Aaron, Robin P., Hallie G., Stefani, Melissa, Karen, Robin F., Kate, Sheryl, Erin, Liz, Hillary, Sloane, Janell, Alan, Amber, Kirstin, Kistie, Diane, Joanne, and Jen for all of your invaluable feedback. Your advice and comments were integral to this book, and all your encouragement helped us reach the finish line.

To Michelle Beadle, we are so honored that you wrote our foreword. We are so flattered by your generous words and are so thankful that you were there for us from the beginning of this journey. Your sense of humor is contagious, and working with you has been a blast.

To Joy Bauer, we are humbled by your support. You are an inspiration to us, as you help so many lead healthier lives. We only hope that a scoop here and there will help us follow in your footsteps.

Our sincere gratitude to Toby Amidor, Joel Harper, and Angie Everhart. You are all the top in your respective fields, and we are so fortunate for your praise.

To Stephen Costello, for your expert advice and thorough guidance. You helped us navigate through this crazy world of publishing and for that we are incredibly grateful.

To Melissa Schiller, for introducing us and realizing our synergy before we did. This book would not have been possible without your matchmaking skills. For both of us, you are the definition of a true friend, and we love you!

Thank you to Brian Marcus and Fred Marcus Photography for being the best in the biz and for making us look good.

We also thank our awesome interns for all of their hard work: Catherine Staffieri, Lauren Sharpe, Ashley Sobel, and Maycee Nicholas. You all have very bright futures ahead of you!

Ilyse

To Hallie: "A dream without a plan is just a wish." Thank you for dreaming that we could do this. It is our combined strength that made our vision a reality. It's amazing how well we work together. Whenever one of us felt like there was no end in sight, the other pushed forward. I couldn't have asked for a better writing partner . . . and friend. This is only the beginning!

To my loving husband, Evan, thank you for believing in me from the beginning. I would not be the woman I am today without your constant support and encouragement.

To Riley and Perri, my two beautiful girls: thank you for your patience and understanding while I wrote. I strive to be a role model for the two of you and show you that you can achieve anything. Girls rule, and I love you!

To my wonderful parents Marlene and Bob: thank you for teaching me that anything can be accomplished if you put your mind to it.

This book would not have been possible without the incredible Barbara Brown, who exhibits such love and concern for my children day after day. And to Hannah Sloane, who spent so many hours entertaining my girls while I snuck in a few hours of writing.

To all of my friends who cheered me on as I opened my practice and wrote this book. You know who you are, and you mean the world to me . . .

And, of course, a huge thank-you to my clients. I would not have had the confidence to write this book without each and every one of you. Thank you for making me a part of your lives and in believing that a life full of health is something we can achieve together.

Hallie

To Ilyse: There is no one else I could have or would have wanted to write this book with. We laughed, we danced, and we cried while working on this book, but it never (okay, almost never) felt like work. This book has been life-changing and you have become more than my coauthor but my life-long friend.

To my husband, Mike. Since the day we met through our first year of marriage, this book has always been on my to-do list. Yet, instead of making me feel guilty, you were my biggest champion. Thank you for your unending support, patience and encouragement. You are my best friend, my true love, and I am honored to be your wife. Love you more.

To my mom, Ronni, and sister, Barrie: Thank you doesn't seem like enough. You have always believed in me and my crazy dreams and have never stopped cheering me on. There are no words to adequately describe how much I love you both and how much you mean to me.

A huge thank-you to the family I was born into and the family I married into for all of your love. You are all so special to me and make me feel like I won the lotto twice.

To all of my friends: thank you for still loving me despite disappearing for long chunks of time while I wrote this book. I am so lucky to have the greatest friends and support system.

To Robin Fromme for being so trustworthy and someone I can always count on. Thanks for all of your help as I know I put on a lot on your shoulders while I had to focus on this book.

To Mel, my mentor and my father. There is not a day that goes by that I don't miss you, but I carry you with me in everything that I do. I was so fortunate to work beside you and see how you so effortlessly combined your passion and intelligence to make a difference in the supplement industry. I was even luckier, though, to have you as my father and am so grateful for all of the life lessons you instilled upon me.

About the Authors

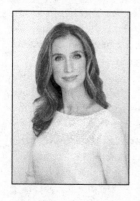

Ilyse Schapiro, MS, RD, CDN, is the Founder & President of Ilyse Schapiro Nutrition, a nutrition counseling and consulting practice. As a nationally recognized expert in the field of nutrition, Ilyse is sought after time and again to offer perspective on nutrition trends and healthy living. Before launching her own private practice, she was a dietitian at Joy Bauer Nutrition and served as a clinical dietitian at the Hospital for Special Surgery. Prior to pursing her graduate degree in clinical nutrition and dietetics from New York University, Ilyse served on the publishing team at Men's Health magazine. Ilyse's work at the award-winning publication inspired her to pursue her personal passion for health and wellness.

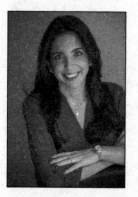

Hallie Rich is proud to be a third generation vitamin industry executive and entrepreneur. She has followed in her family's lauded footsteps as an innovative force in that industry with the creation of the award winning alternaVites vitamin and mineral brand of melt-in-your-mouth powdered vitamins for both adults and children. She has redefined how people take their daily vitamins, especially for the immense portion of the population who cannot swallow vitamins and for those looking for alternative options for their children. She is regarded as a pioneer and expert in her field and was recently elected to the Board of Directors of The Natural Products Association East. Hallie received her BA with honors from the University of Michigan. She is also the co-founder of Rich in Love, a charity that raises money for cancer research and prevention programs.